Going Green
Before You Conceive

Revitalize Fertility, Radiate During
Pregnancy, Birth and Beyond

Wendie Aston

BALBOA.
PRESS
A DIVISION OF HAY HOUSE

Cover design and photograph by William Graf
Author photograph by Bradford Rogne
Editing by Judie Harvey

www.greenonthescene.blogspot.com

Balboa Press books may be ordered through booksellers or by contacting:

Balboa Press
A Division of Hay House
1663 Liberty Drive
Bloomington, IN 47403
www.balboapress.com
1 (877) 407-4847

Print information available on the last page.

ISBN: 978-1-5043-4897-3 (sc)
ISBN: 978-1-5043-4898-0 (e)

Library of Congress Control Number: 2016905617

Balboa Press rev. date: 10/20/2016

For my greatest loves, Brooke, Harley and Zander.

CONTENTS

PREFACE

My journey to parenthood was not an easy one. My husband and I did not conceive our first child until after we were married for five years and I was 35. I had several health issues ranging from endometriosis, hyperprolactinemia, hypothyroid, gluten intolerance, small fiber neuropathy and candida overgrowth. What no one ever said was that each of these health issues can affect conception if not treated properly. Also, being told I was in pre-menopause at 33 didn't help our confidence about becoming parents.

I thought my diet was healthy at the time. My husband is a trained chef and made most of our meals. Perhaps I consumed too much sugar? Maybe the years of using birth control pills threw my hormones out of control? Or maybe the toxic chemicals I exposed myself to during DIY home renovations were taking their toll? Whatever the reason, I found that changing our routine and adopting GREEN habits and an organic lifestyle helped us succeed in becoming parents.

Our first pregnancy happened when we were not expecting it. After only one month of taking Cytomel (which is T3 hormone) and Nature Throid (natural hormone replacement) to treat my hypothyroidism, I became pregnant. I was already on a gluten free diet and eating organic as much as possible so that may have helped. We had been transitioning into a more holistic lifestyle at that point so what we were doing provided the right combination for conception. My husband and I were beyond shocked when we found out we were expecting a baby.

Greening our lives was a slow process that started with organic eating and then eliminating my harmful makeup and personal care products that throw hormones off balance. I was constantly researching new ways of living a greener healthier life since I seemed to be sensitive to fragrances and synthetic chemicals found in many of these beauty products.

From then I went to detoxing my household cleaning routine. Getting a headache after cleaning the bathroom didn't seem to make sense to me. The chemicals in the conventional cleaners I was inhaling were making me sick.

Changing to natural products for the home like vinegar for cleaning, latex pillows and mattresses, using non-toxic cooking equipment, and remodeling with non-toxic paints and products easily followed. While this process can be overwhelming, my misdiagnoses and years of infertility were more so. If there was a non-toxic option out there, I was sure to find it!

When it became a challenge to get pregnant a second time and suffering two miscarriages, we turned to alternative methods to help with conception. I also had fallen into a rut of consuming too much sugar again and had to fine tune my diet. I began using acupuncture and herbs to boost fertility in addition to my healthy eating and living. Using Chinese medicine to treat fertility seemed to work for us and we were pregnant again.

The third baby was the easiest to conceive at the age of 40! Now I had pulled out all of the stops in wanting to try for a boy with an alkaline diet and timing of sex. We also incorporated feng shui, fertility massage, yoga, and acupuncture, herbs and prayer. All of our efforts worked better than we envisioned.

The GREENER our lives became, the healthier and happier we felt. We also knew that having a GREEN pregnancy, birth and upbringing were something our family would embrace. I researched all of the healthiest baby products on the market when I was expecting our first child and selected only those that I believed to be the safest. Our birth plans even included hypnobirthing, an excellent method to birthing also without the use of drugs.

The greatest compliment to your mission of becoming a parent, is the belief that it can be done. Whether you are already a parent or plan to become one, it is my sincere desire this book will guide you on a healthy journey to become as GREEN as you can *BEFORE* you conceive.

ACKNOWLEGEMENTS

Bill Graf for capturing my pregnancy and
designing the cover I envisioned

Judie Harvey for working miracles with
words in such a delicate time frame

Kathy Shamoun for teaching me that a
natural drug free birth is possible

Pailin Winotaka for supporting me throughout
my pregnancies in all stages

Ann Boroch for teaching me to eat healthier
and eliminate my Candida overgrowth

Dr. Boris Katz for determining exactly what my body needed

Catalina Rivera for her knowledge and support

Pamela Rich for sharing her love of Young Living Essential oils

Misty Crouch, Lindsay Hall, Kelli Kirkland, for encouraging
me to start my blog, and continue on this journey of writing

Stony Brook University Midwives for their
support of natural childbirth

My husband, Matt, for his love and support throughout this journey

CHAPTER ONE: WHY GO GREEN?

When couples decide they want to have a baby, most simply long for a healthy child. Women want to conceive right away and have a happy, healthy pregnancy, too. If you want to conceive a healthy child and feel great during your pregnancy my first suggestion is to go green before you conceive. "Green" brings to mind different definitions and connotations: non-toxic, safe for the environment, and healthy. It is also associated with the fourth or heart chakra, which symbolizes health, harmony, creativity, abundance, and nature. Going green, as it relates to health, can be one of the best steps you take in your life. If green is associated with abundance and nature, it makes sense that we can all have many children naturally if we live a "green" and healthy life. Most importantly, being green can change the way a life is formed in the womb.

The amount of toxic substances we come in contact with every day is alarming. Imagine how this affects our ability to reproduce. In Sandra Steingraber's book *Having Faith* she writes: "If the world's environment is contaminated, so too is the ecosystem of a mother's body. If a mother's body is contaminated, so too is the child who inhabits it." As an ecologist, author, and mother, Steingraber knows the importance of living a green life when trying to procreate. When we choose to have children, we should really think about what is going into our bodies from all angles, including the food we eat, the air we breathe, and what we touch. If our bodies contain toxins, so do our babies. Babies born today can have over 200 industrial chemicals found in their umbilical cord blood.[1] If we can take steps to reduce or eliminate this, it must be done.

By starting with small steps you can detoxify your home, diet, beauty routine, cleaning routine, and almost every aspect of your life. Doing this in my own life made a great impact on my ability to conceive naturally. After reading a magazine article on the dangers of chemicals in my makeup, I tossed out EVERYTHING and purchased makeups that were free of chemicals and all natural. This also included replacing my shampoos and moisturizers. Anything that went on my skin became truly free of anything toxic that would disrupt my hormones. All of the cleaners that I had bought in bulk had to go as well and were replaced with non-toxic options.

The amount of time, energy, and money put into raising a child is enormous. Giving your child the greatest advantage by creating healthy eggs and sperm is one of the best things you can do for him or her.

Most people do not realize it takes approximately three months for eggs to mature for ovulation, while sperm is ready in seventy-two days. When you think of everything your body could be exposed to in the months leading up to conception, it makes sense to take the time to learn how going green before you conceive can improve your reproductive health. Making changes in your life to go green can result in better health for you overall, and it can help sustain our environment as well. Most importantly it can give you the best chance at producing the healthiest sperm and eggs and, eventually, a healthy, happy baby.

An all-natural approach to pregnancy can be the least invasive and least expensive. Years ago, conceiving a child was not a problem for the majority of the population. Today some have success without changing their lives at all, while others struggle for months and even years before they become parents. Some couples are told they have "unexplained infertility," which is not very comforting since most people expect doctors to have answers. While there are numerous fertility clinics trying to help couples become parents, I often wonder how many couples could be helped, simply by making some greener lifestyle choices.

A lot of couples also have recurrent miscarriages. Others carry a child to the third trimester and then have pre-term labor, resulting in numerous complications, for example immature lungs, which can lead to chronic respiratory issues. Even when couples do succeed in getting pregnant, their child may develop autism, ADHD, allergies, and other medical conditions that can be traced back to prenatal care and environment. The statistics are troublesome.

While we cannot explain exactly why these things happen, we do know that exposure to toxins can wreak havoc on the body and babies in utero. The significant number of toxic chemicals that we are exposed to either through our food supply or from things we come in contact with on a daily basis cannot be ignored. Consumers are not protected from harmful chemicals in everyday products. We must do our own research before buying if we want to eliminate toxins from our lives. Often untested in everyday products, these toxins are affecting our health whether we realize it or not.

Even the way that women give birth has changed dramatically. What was once a natural process has become everything but. The percentage of women having a C-section as opposed to birthing naturally has skyrocketed. Now about one in three women give birth via C-section according to Childbirthconnection.org. In 1965 the national average was just 4.5 percent for women who had C-sections. Inductions and C-sections are scheduled like making an appointment to get your hair cut. Conception and birth should not be this difficult or this medicalized. Despite all of the medical advances we have access to when it comes to childbearing and childbirth, we still have a lot of work to do to make things safer for mother and child.

When we decide to conceive, many of us do not think about the environmental impact that one more human will have. Each person affects the planet by the choices he or she makes in everyday life. While everyone has a different path to parenthood, giving your child a safe, healthy environment to begin their life is the best option for any parent-to-be. If you continue that green lifestyle throughout childhood with the right food and environmental choices, you can have the healthiest kid on the block. If you make an effort to live an eco-friendly life, and show your children how to do this as well, your efforts to "green the planet" that God created will make a more sustainable future for us all.

I'll show you that this is easier than you think!

CHAPTER TWO: GET IN THE BEST OF HEALTH FOR YOU AND YOUR BABY

When you decide it is time to try and conceive, there are steps you can take to increase your odds of having a healthy baby. First of all, you should get a full check-up with your health care provider—whether it be an OB-GYN or a midwife. If you don't have one, choosing one will depend on what type of birth you envision: a home birth, a birthing center, a hospital, or other alternatives. "The Business of Being Born" is an excellent, guiding film that will give you insight on the birthing process and help you make the proper decision as a couple on what type of caregiver you want on your parenthood journey. If you have any pre-existing medical conditions such as diabetes, high blood pressure, an autoimmune disease like multiple sclerosis or health factors that make you high risk, you will need an ob-gyn to ensure the safest possible process.

While C-section rates are higher for OB-GYNs, midwives do not usually handle high-risk pregnancies. However, if you are healthy, able, and dreaming of a natural vaginal birth with little intervention, midwives are not only less clinical in demeanor but also have lower rates of C-sections.

It might be tempting to say *but I'm healthy—I don't need all this fuss.* Think of it this way: Would you plan a cross-country drive before getting your car tuned up? Having and raising a child is one of the most important journeys you will take in your life, and it's important to make sure that your body is ready for the trip. There are more and more undiagnosed issues that affect a woman's ability to conceive, such as hypothyroidism, celiac disease or gluten intolerance, PCOS (Polycystic Ovarian Syndrome), HP (hyperprolactinemia—high prolactin level causing discharge from nipples), pre-diabetes, gene defects, endometriosis, candida and many others.

Some fertility issues can be easily fixed by changing your diet. "You are what you eat" speaks volumes when it comes to fertility. By maintaining a healthy, nutrient-rich diet that is low in sugar with fertility-boosting foods, you are sure to supercharge your eggs. In extreme instances, you may need medication or even surgery. Anyone who has suffered from infertility issues can tell you that discovering a crushing surprise late in the game can be devastating. It is far better to rule out every possible delay early on. Remember that you are not alone in this journey! Your partner should be getting a full work-up too to ensure sperm health. Getting proper check-ups from someone you trust with a more natural approach to childbearing may help you avoid complications and unnecessary medications.

You also want to make sure you are at a proper weight and have your blood sugar levels under control. Your ideal waist size should be your height divided by two. According to Dr. Margaret Ashwell, former science director of the British Nutrition Foundation, waist size is more important than overall weight in detecting high blood pressure, diabetes and risk for heart attacks and strokes.[2]

Testing blood sugar levels has become increasingly important with the rising occurrences of pre-diabetes, a strong indicator for likely gestational diabetes in pregnancy. It is of utmost importance to have a balanced diet before pregnancy and make sure your sugar intake is low. Because more and more Americans are consuming high glycemic foods—foods high in carbs and sugar—at an increasing rate, the "skinny-fat" phenomenon has emerged. "Dr. Daniel Neides, medical director at Cleveland Clinic's Wellness Institute says: "On the outside they look incredibly healthy, but on the inside they're a wreck."[3]

These individuals look healthy on the outside, but are besieged with the blood sugar levels of someone who is medically obese. If you are having trouble controlling sugar intake, you can learn more from Dr. Mark Hyman's books, *The Blood Sugar Solution 10-Day Detox Diet* or

The Blood Sugar Solution. Our diets contain way too much sugar, refined flour, and soda. It is best to cut these items out before pregnancy so as not to develop major problems down the road. In mild cases, blood sugar levels can be controlled strictly by a disciplined diet rather than popping pills. Some medications, like glyburide and metformin, have not been thoroughly tested for use during pregnancy, although some doctors still prescribe them to women who wish to conceive.[4] If you read all of the fine print, the side effects are often worse than the actual symptoms you may be having. Diet is key for blood sugar regulation, not medication.

Thyroid

Tests should also include a full blood panel and testing for thyroid levels, which include TSH, T4 and T3, reverse T3, TgAb antibodies, TPO and maybe prolactin levels. One common issue women face is undiagnosed hypothyroidism. This can make it difficult to conceive and lead to miscarriage and other problems. In addition to lab work, another way to test for hypothyroidism is by charting your basal body temperature. You will need a basal body thermometer which is different that a regular thermometer. It senses your temperature at rest with more accuracy to 1/10th of a degree. This also will help you plan your conception time. It is best to put the basal body temperature thermometer under your pillow or in your nightstand so you test before you get out of bed. Temperature should be taken at the same time each morning and put into a chart, easily found online. If temperatures are too low—according to some practitioners, 97.6 or lower before ovulation—and you experience symptoms of sluggishness, sensitivity to cold, depression, weight gain, dry skin, thinning or loss of hair, loss of the outer third of eyebrow, heavy periods, hoarseness, or an enlarged neck (goiter), you may have hypothyroidism. If you are diagnosed, further treatment is required before conceiving.

An endocrinologist or naturopath can help get your thyroid levels under control. Not all doctors follow the same guidelines for blood levels, so if you do have symptoms and a low temperature, seek a second opinion and be sure to test T3, T4, and TSH levels. Again, not all doctors test for everything. You need to ask for specific tests so you know exactly what is going on with your body. In addition, some people have trouble converting T4 to T3 and may need a medication like Cytomel, which is T3 rather than just the medication Synthroid, which is T4. Tirosint is also T4 and free of gluten and colorings. There are also natural options like Nature Throid. Everyone's body will react differently. Not all treatments work the same for everyone, and it may take a few months to see what works for you.

Celiac Disease and Gluten Intolerance

There is also a link between celiac disease, gluten intolerance, and infertility. If you have symptoms of irritable bowel, diarrhea, constipation, bloating, abdominal pain, gynecological issues, skin rash, weight loss, joint pain, tingling in the hands and feet, anemia, or brain fog, you may want to investigate this further before you begin trying to conceive. For me, *Celiac Disease: A Hidden Epidemic* by Peter H. R. Green, MD, the Director of the Celiac Disease Center at Columbia University, was a great eye opener. Patients with celiac disease may in fact have thyroid issues as well. Having celiac puts you at an increased risk of developing autoimmune diseases such as hypothyroid. "People with celiac disease are nearly four times more likely to develop an autoimmune thyroid condition" according to celiac central.org. Talk about conception becoming challenging if you have both! Celiac disease can wreak havoc on the small intestine while gluten intolerance will present the same symptoms but stop short of organ damage. Many women who are diagnosed with unexplained infertility find out later that they indeed have celiac disease or gluten intolerance. "One study conducted by physicians at Thomas Jefferson University Hospital in Philadelphia found that the rate of recurrent spontaneous abortion (RSAB) and infertility in celiac disease patients is at least four times higher than the general population. They suggested that patients who experience unexplained infertility or RSAB should be screened for celiac disease."[5] Even women with PCOS (Polycystic Ovarian Syndrome) are encouraged to begin eating a gluten-free diet to restore their missed periods and fertility.

Celiac disease also contributes to the poor quality of male sperm and their motility, so be sure to ask your husband how his digestion and overall health is before you begin your path to parenthood. If you find you have an issue with gluten or wheat, a gluten-free diet is a relatively simple solution. While it is difficult at first, your healthy baby will be well worth it. There are more and more options available today for those that must or want to go gluten-free. Just be aware that some of the substitute flours can have a high glycemic effect. Cookies are still cookies! Cakes are still cakes. Just because you are going gluten-free doesn't give you carte blanche to binge on every boxed or baked gluten-free item on the market. Keep in mind that many of these items are not organic. Finding organic and non-GMO gluten-free items can be a challenge at first, but there are some great options out there.

Gluten-Free Non-GMO Products (not all Gluten Free Products are Organic)

Bread: RUDI's, Canyon Bakehouse, Amy's Organic Sandwich Rounds (can also be used as pizza crust), Bob's Gluten-Free Grain Bread Mix, All Purpose Flour

Crackers: RW Garcia Crackers, Mediterranean Snacks Lentil Crackers

Pasta: Black Bean, Mung Bean, Ancient Harvest Quinoa Pasta

You can also make your own gluten-free bread and baked goods with various flours, such as garbanzo, almond flour or almond meal, and buckwheat. Even slightly more complicated meals like homemade gluten-free gnocchi are easy to make. A lot of the frozen or premade gluten free options contain soy or canola oil, which should be avoided. These oils are less than satisfactory and should not be part of your diet. Soy is a GMO, contains goitrogens which are bad for thyroid function and acts like estrogen in the body. Canola, another top GMO, becomes rancid when heated.

Polycystic Ovarian Syndrome (PCOS)

If you find yourself with missing or irregular periods, acne, excessive hair growth, or obesity, you may have PCOS. You may even have cysts on your ovaries, which is one of the more severe symptoms. The less severe symptoms you may overlook but should be aware of if you are trying to conceive. The cause of PCOS is unknown, but there are options for treatment in the traditional medical realm as well as with strict diets. *The PCOS Diet Plan: A Natural Approach to Health for Women with Polycystic Ovarian Syndrome* by Hillary Wright is a great help for charting out what you can do without resorting to medication. Some practitioners, like PCOS Nutrition Center Founder Angela Grassi, suggest eliminating gluten as well as. Grassi discusses this in the book *The PCOS Nutrition Center Cookbook*. If you have gluten sensitivity, it can cause chronic inflammation. Women with PCOS most likely already have chronic inflammation, so eating gluten should be a no-no. There are women who have had PCOS and changed their diet alone and became pregnant within a couple months. You can find blogs and success stories all over the Internet. There may not be medical statistics to back this up currently, but I know someone who has a new baby after suffering from PCOS and simply changed her diet. No medical intervention was needed for them. Let food be thy medicine, as they say!

High Levels of Prolactin

Hyperprolactinemia—when your prolactin hormone levels are higher than normal—is another fertility issue that some women face. The hormone prolactin is present during pregnancy and helps women produce breast milk. Hyperprolactinemia causes nipple discharge, loss of period, and may even prohibit you from ovulating, leading to infertility. Causes range from pituitary tumors to hypothyroidism, stress, breast stimulation, and even the use of certain medications. Depending on your situation, hopefully you can get your prolactin levels under control and ovulate without a problem. My own prolactin issue started for me soon after I was prescribed a birth control pill with high levels of progestin in it—another reason I believe natural family planning is better than throwing your body chemistry into confusion with synthetic hormones. I was able to use the medication cabergoline at a minimal dose for one pregnancy and acupuncture alone for the other pregnancy.

Endometriosis

Endometriosis—one of the major causes of infertility—is extremely painful for some women, while barely presenting any symptoms in others. The most common are painful periods, pain with intercourse (that doesn't help the baby-making process), pain with bowel movements or urination, heavy periods or bleeding between periods, fatigue, other symptoms associated with irritable bowel syndrome, and of course, infertility. You can understand why this is such a hard condition to diagnose; the symptoms overlap with many other possible conditions and misdiagnoses are common.

Endometriosis is defined as the growth of endometrial cells outside of the uterus. These cells normally grow in the uterus each month, preparing the body for pregnancy. When the pregnancy is not achieved, they are released by having a period. Cells can grow on the ovaries, fallopian tubes, intestines, and all over the pelvic region, making conception difficult in some cases.

The only sure way to diagnose endometriosis properly is with a laparoscopy, where small incisions are made in the pelvic region and the doctor can see if tissues appear where they should not. Sometimes tissue is removed and biopsied for confirmation. Talk with your doctor to see if this is a necessary procedure. An operation may reveal few signs of endometriosis or a major case. Either way, it can most likely be removed during the laparoscopy, and you could begin trying to conceive just months later. While it is usually an outpatient procedure, it is still surgery where you will be medicated and have a few stitches and incisions in one or more areas of the abdomen. A detox protocol from the medication may be in order after you have the procedure, especially if you chose heavy-duty pain medication.

Be aware that endometriosis can reoccur, since it is fueled by estrogen found in both the body itself and in beauty products and food. However, certain diet guidelines can keep it at bay. First, eliminate wheat, dairy (including whey and casein), soy (which is estrogenic), caffeine, saturated fat, and hormones found in meat (cutting out red meat entirely would be even a greater help). Avoiding alcohol (which can also raise levels of estrogen), sugar, fried food, preservatives, and additives is recommended. Eat organic when possible, increase your intake of omega-3 fatty acids, and drink red raspberry leaf tea to help reduce cramping. The list of what you need to eliminate might seem intimidating, but if you're in pain, you'll find it an easy transition once you start experiencing relief.

MTHFR Gene

One of the newest complications to watch out for is an obscure gene mutation, which many women are not aware of—and, in some cases, neither are their doctors. The MTHFR gene (*Methylenetetrahydrofolate reductase*) gene, known as MTHFR C677T causes the body to improperly use up the folic acid supplements that help prevent birth defects during pregnancy. "For one in four people, this is a serious reality and, if left undiagnosed, may lead to a variety of pregnancy-related issues including, difficulties conceiving, unexplained infertility, elevated homocysteine levels, Down Syndrome, autism, preeclampsia, postpartum depression, the development of chronic depression, and even recurrent miscarriages."[6] This gene also plays many other important roles in the body than can affect all sorts of functions, even the ability to process toxins. It also can cause elevated homocysteine levels, which can trigger a miscarriage. While not everyone will want or need this test, it is good to be aware of, if you are sensitive to chemical smells, fragrances, or are easily affected by environmental toxins. Do you get headaches or nausea from being exposed to certain smells or synthetic fragrances? Do you suffer from IBS, chronic fatigue, migraines, depression, addictions, fibromyalgia, or blood clots? If so, you may want to talk to your doctor and see if you are one of the growing number of women who are being diagnosed with this gene expression or the A1298C mutation since it can make your body more sensitive to daily toxins and in some cases make conceiving a bit more challenging. Check out MTHFR.net for more information.

Candida

Candida is also known as a yeast overgrowth. It can affect men and women to varying degrees. You have a greater risk at developing it if you have a diet high in sugar and carbs, drink alcohol, eat fermented foods, take oral contraceptives, have taken antibiotics, and have a stressful lifestyle. That sounds like most of us may have it or be at risk for developing it.

Women who have yeast overgrowth experience frequent yeast infections. This can be especially true if they have been on birth control pills for years. It can also contribute to hormonal imbalances and maybe even endometriosis.

Left untreated, it can cause a variety of symptoms other than just intestinal issues. If you suspect you have it, get in under control before trying to conceive. Many doctors do not test for candida, but you can learn more at www.annboroch.com or read the book *The Candida Cure*, by Ann Boroch, CNC. She is a naturopath who healed herself of multiple sclerosis and has been free of symptoms for 20 years.

Oral Hygiene

In addition to taking care of your body prior to conception, you also must take care of your oral health. Before the three-month window of egg and sperm maturation, you will want to see the dentist to have a cleaning and take care of any dental repair that may be needed. During pregnancy you will also want to have at least one or two cleanings. No

X-rays! Our oral hygiene or lack thereof during pregnancy can lead to other issues such as swollen gums and excess bleeding or gingivitis. You may notice your gums bleed more when you are pregnant. Making sure plaque is removed by a proper cleaning at the dentist will help lessen bleeding.

During pregnancy, there is also a chance you may develop tumors or granulomas on the gums, which will go away after pregnancy in most cases. They are harmless red or purple bumps that usually appear during the second trimester. Brushing twice a day with something like an electric toothbrush and regularly flossing are the best defenses against dental problems. According to research there is also a link between gingivitis and low birth weight babies and pre-term labor. Even if you are cavity-free and have white teeth, schedule a visit to the dentist prior to conception and at least once during pregnancy to help eliminate any risks. It is also in your best interest to find a holistic dentist who does not use mercury fillings in the office and is a member of the Holistic Dental Association. Eliminating exposure to any toxins, even if you are not the one getting the fillings, is so important during this time.

Eat Organic

Now that you have your blood tests done, a physical exam, and trip to the dentist you may think now is the time to try and make a baby if you are given a clean bill of health. Hold off a bit and for good reason. Since it takes approximately three months for eggs to mature for ovulation while it takes around 72 days for sperm to mature you want to make sure you are in the clear of any environmental toxins and have a healthy diet before you begin trying to conceive. Sometimes an unhealthy egg or sperm can be released and fertilization will not occur due to many outside factors. Or sadly, fertilization does occur but the baby is unhealthy resulting in a miscarriage or birth defects. What this means is that you and your partner should be eating a healthy organic diet and eliminate exposure to environmental factors for at least three months prior to trying. This includes if you have been taking a prescription medication or have had a severe illness that you or your partner are recovering from, or lastly engaged in heavy drinking or smoking. What goes in your body or what you breathe before conception can affect egg and sperm health. You want to be in top shape as if you are preparing for a marathon. Think of it as a nine-and-a-half month (or longer, depending on how long it takes to conceive) marathon.

So, have at least three months of healthy, organic, non-toxic, drug-free, smoke-free living before trying to make a baby! Do not forget to have a proper check-up for both you and your partner. Some of you may get pregnant without much effort, hooray! Do not stress out that you didn't follow the three-month protocol. Continue with your healthy lifestyle, stay clear of toxins, and enjoy the pregnancy.

CHAPTER THREE: GREEN YOUR DIET IN MORE WAYS THAN ONE

There are several areas in which you can and should "green" your life before actually trying to conceive. We have all heard the phrase *You are what you eat.* Be aware: Your baby is what you eat, too. The first step is to take a look at your diet as a couple. It is not all just about what the woman eats. Men also need to consider what their daily diet is. Avoid fast food, fried foods, sugar, processed foods, anything with food coloring added, alcohol, soda, and caffeine. If you incorporate a healthy diet well before you become pregnant, and then continue with this diet throughout your pregnancy, you are less likely to have health issues. With a good eating plan firmly in place, you may also be able to better control the urge to eat unnecessary or unhealthy choices during your pregnancy.

Some women experience excess weight gain because they feel that it is all right to binge eat when they are pregnant. You really do not need to eat double the amounts of food! Eating for two does not mean eating twice the amount. Some women also feel that they should give in to *every craving*! While some cravings may mean you are lacking something nutritionally, giving in to ice cream every night can lead to gestational diabetes. Sure, there will be times when you feel you have to give in to a craving or you are at a party where there are no other options. Try to make these occurrences the exception to the rule.

What you eat before you conceive has a major effect on the baby's DNA and how he or she develops. Most people start to change their diet when they find out they are pregnant. As I mentioned, this actually is better if it is done at least three months before conceiving to create healthy eggs and sperm. My advice is to be aware, use common sense, and make sure you are eating organic and non-GMO foods as often as possible.

The Right Balance

You may be wondering how green you should be eating. If you are thinking I am going to recommend a vegetarian or vegan diet, I am not. There are some women who can sustain a pregnancy on these types of diets and feel great doing so. However, if you look throughout history, man has eaten meat—women, too! Many cultures thrive on different foods, including meats, and have no trouble conceiving. There are a lot of necessary fats and nutrients needed by the body that we can only get from meat. Though there are alternatives for the determined, not everyone's body will accept alternatives.

I believe it is far more difficult to sustain a healthy pregnancy without the necessary fats and nutrients found only in meats. Based on the research of Dr. Weston A. Price, some women do better on a diet higher in fats, meats, dairy, and lower in carbs and sugar.[7] This means eating full-fat foods, not low-fat. Please know that if you have any disorders, such as PCOS or endometriosis, this advice does not apply to you. If you are challenged with these conditions, you will want to avoid an overload of dairy and red meat, since these foods can cause or exacerbate these particular health issues.

A Word About GMOs and Eating Organic

Next, you should avoid genetically modified foods or organisms, otherwise known as GMOs. These foods comprise about 75 percent of the food at the grocery store. Instead choose non-GMO Project-verified or 100 percent organic products. The research shows how dramatically GMOs affect animals, increasing the likelihood of infertility as well as a whole host of other health issues. Jeffrey Smith's film *Genetic Roulette* illustrates effectively why it is in our interest to avoid GMOs.

This is not to be taken lightly since we're still in the dark about the full ramifications for our genes and the future of our genetic makeup.

Most Common GMOs to Avoid

Soybeans
Soy products (soy oil, soy protein, soy isolate, vegetable oil)
Corn products (corn, corn flour, corn masa, corn meal, canola oil)
Cottonseed oil
Flax products (flax seeds and oil)
Rice products (rice, rice flour, rice milk)
Alfalfa
Papaya
Zucchini
Yellow Summer Squash
Sugar Beets (including sugar processed from these crops)
Sugar (corn, fructose, sucrose)
Apples and recently Potatoes

Other possible GMOs include plums, peas, radicchio, tomatoes, cantaloupe, sweet pepper, tobacco, salmon, and pork products containing omega-3 fatty acids!

Pesticides from non-organic food can travel through the umbilical cord to your unborn baby. Babies are increasingly born with high levels of toxins found in their umbilical cord blood. One way to reduce exposure is to eat organic whenever possible. Consult the Environmental Working Group's (EWG.org) Dirty Dozen and Clean Fifteen lists when shopping for produce so you can avoid the fruits and vegetables most prone to contamination.

As an expectant couple, you should be extra careful in examining labels and choosing organic, pasture-raised, non-GMO proteins, such as beef, bison, chicken, dairy, eggs, pork, and lamb. Unless they are raised organically, these animals are most likely ingesting GMOs. They also may be injected with hormones or antibiotics. Do not be fooled by the words "all natural." That does not mean the meat is hormone or GMO-free—it is an unregulated term that companies are free to use on their labels. If you buy from a CSA or local farm, you will know how the animals are raised and treated. Getting meats from factory farms should be avoided, and unfortunately that is what is in the majority of the supermarkets.

Seafood

There are studies that imply you should not consume any seafood while you are pregnant, due to the fact that most of it is riddled with toxins from our poisoned oceans, lake, and ponds. Mercury is the biggest culprit and is most commonly found in ahi tuna, shark, king mackerel, marlin, orange roughy, tilefish, and swordfish. These fish have the highest levels of mercury and should be avoided altogether three months prior to conception, throughout pregnancy, and when breastfeeding. Chilean sea bass, bluefish, grouper, Spanish or Gulf mackerel, albacore canned tuna, and yellowfin tuna are safer, but still contain enough mercury that the American Pregnancy Association recommends you consume them no more than three times a month. To be on the safe side, I would suggest eating them even less often or not at all.

Even small amounts of mercury can be damaging to your health and to the health of a developing fetus. I experienced this personally when I had mercury poisoning after college because I was eating canned tuna three times a week. I did not have any mercury fillings that could cause high levels. The only source the doctor could find was from my diet. I needed weeks-long chelation therapy to remove the mercury from my body.

The fish that contain lower levels of mercury are striped and black bass, carp, Alaskan cod (beware of radiation levels though), white Pacific croaker, Pacific and Atlantic halibut, lobster, mahi mahi, monkfish, freshwater perch, sablefish, skate, snapper, sea trout, canned chunk tuna, and skipjack tuna. Alaskan and West Coast seafood spanning the Pacific fishing grounds to Japan have high toxicity levels of radiation due to Japan's Fukushima Nuclear Reactor leak, so caution should be taken with any catch from that region. Though these fish are documented as being safer to eat, there is no way to verify what toxins they may be ingesting—the same toxins that will end up in our bodies and our babies—so I prefer to consume no more than once a month or not at all.

Lastly, the fish with the lowest levels of mercury are anchovies, butterfish, catfish, clam, domestic crab, crawfish, crayfish, croaker, flounder, haddock, hake, herring, North Atlantic and chub mackerel, mullet, oysters, ocean perch, place, canned and fresh salmon (avoid farmed), sardines, scallops, American shad, shrimp, sole, calamari or squid, tilapia, freshwater trout, whitefish, and whiting. For these relatively safe fish, I would recommend a 6-oz serving a week or every other week if you have a craving.

Other than mercury levels, the major issue with fish and seafood is that it's so difficult to source their origin. Also, some seafood are "bottom feeders," including shellfish, like lobster, shrimp, and crab as well as fleshy fish, including catfish, cod, flounder, halibut.[8] These fish are called bottom feeders because they consume whatever is on the bottom of the ocean. Eating them means that you and your unborn baby are also ingesting whatever matter is at the bottom of the sea, including oil, chemicals, and toxins. Thailand, China, and other countries with bad environmental track records have toxins that will saturate the atmosphere, the groundwater, and the coasts—wild seafood in particular from these regions can be dangerous, and even farm-raised fish can be questionable.

Regulations vary wildly across the world, and we don't know what the fish have been exposed to when we purchase it. There are even variations domestically. For example, if you buy local catfish, is the pond or stream that it came from riddled with toxins from a nearby manufacturing plant? Unless you truly know where your food is coming from, I would use caution. Sometimes stores or fish shops have even been known to mislabel fish purposefully so they can charge more money for a particular fish. Buyer beware!

Because of all of these factors, I was extremely careful during all my pregnancies with fish consumption. I ate anchovies, sardines, shrimp from a U.S. fishery, wild salmon, wild cod, or calamari and scallops, in moderation and occasionally when I dined out. I eliminated Alaskan and Gulf seafood altogether. There are simply too many unknowns when it comes to seafood, and it's not worth risking your health or your baby's.

Fruits and Vegetables

Next, take a look at how much produce you are getting into your diet. Is your plate a colorful variety? Are you eating fruits and vegetables that are in season? Getting the proper amount of nutrients from fresh vegetables will boost your health and that of your eggs, sperm, and your baby on the way. Colorful vegetables will give you an array of vitamins and minerals with each meal. If you are following Chinese medicine practices for eating to conceive, you will want to cook your vegetables to some degree by roasting, blanching, or sautéing. If cooking in water, do not over-boil, because this causes the food to lose many of its nutrients. Try a variety of veggies and try to eat food that is in season. As I mentioned earlier, always choose organic and non-GMO whenever possible.

Limit the amount of white potatoes (and related products such as French fries) that you eat, since these do not have the best nutrients and can raise blood sugar levels. It is best to go for the greens before you conceive! This can include spinach, kale, salads of all types (except iceberg, which is less nutritious), cucumbers, broccoli, Swiss chard, and even dandelion greens! There are so many other delicious, colorful vegetables to choose from, such as varieties of squash, sweet potatoes, peppers, tomatoes, pumpkins, radishes, eggplant and more. The more you add variety to your foods, the more nutrients you will give your body.

Nightshade vegetables are those that grow at night. They include white potatoes, tomatoes, eggplant, and peppers. For some people, they cause an aching or burning feeling in your hands or feet after eating or the next day. Not all people are sensitive to nightshade vegetables, but if you are consuming them and have aches and pains, you may want to eliminate them and see if symptoms subside. The nutrients from these are great, but if they cause inflammation for you, it is best to avoid them.

Don't forget about onions, garlic, bok choy, cabbage, Brussels sprouts, and any vegetables you have not tried. Variety is great for your diet and will give you new things to cook if you have been on a limited diet. Adding in new vegetables will boost the nutrients you receive and make dinners interesting!

Fruit is great in the summer when there is such a wonderful variety to choose from at farmers markets or your local grocer. Fruit is the best snack if you are having a craving for sugar, and much healthier for you than products with processed sugar. A bowl of berries beats a plate of cookies. Be sure to have a fruit high in vitamin C, since it can improve fertility and hormone levels in women and improve sperm quality in men. It is best to choose organic, of course, but if it is not available to you, use the Environmental Working Group's list to prioritize when you should invest in organic and when you can be more relaxed about buying organic.

EWGs Dirty Dozen *Plus* List

Choose organic for:

Apples

Strawberries

Blueberries

Grapes

Celery

Peaches

Spinach

Sweet Bell Peppers

Nectarines

Cucumbers

Cherry Tomatoes

Snap Peas

Potatoes

Hot Peppers

Kale

EWGs Clean 15
(contain fewer pesticides)

Avocados

Sweet corn

Pineapples

Cabbage

Sweet peas (frozen)

Onions

Asparagus

Mangoes

Papayas

Kiwi

Eggplant

Grapefruit

Cantaloupe (domestic)

Cauliflower

Sweet potatoes

Grains and Healthy Grain Alternatives

Are you gluten-free? It's possible that you should be. Like nightshade vegetables, grains do not agree with all people. They are higher in carbs and can spike blood sugar at times. See how your body reacts when trying new grains. There are a lot of gluten-free options that are healthier and more nutrient-dense than wheat and gluten products.

- Quinoa is a great gluten free choice and can be used like rice. It is high in protein, nutrient rich, contains anti-inflammatory phytonutrients, and is easy to prepare, too. Quinoa can last in the refrigerator for a few days and be made into different meals. It can be eaten hot or cold, served as a quinoa salad, mixed with your favorite veggies, or as a side dish with butter and herbs.
- Rice is another popular food for many. It can be both a good and a bad choice, depending on certain factors. In recent years there has been cause for concern about arsenic levels in rice. Brown rice contains more arsenic than white. Rice grown in the U.S. has more arsenic than rice from other countries. Basmati and jasmine rice are thought to be the safer options. If you have been consuming lots of rice, try not to worry. You can detox in an Epsom salt bath to remove the trace amounts of arsenic that might be in your system. While it is always better to be cautious, when compared to the levels of mercury found in fish, trace amounts of arsenic are not life-threatening. Also, be aware that if you are going gluten-free, rice is often a substitute for wheat in prepared or boxed foods, so you may be consuming more rice than the average person. Read the labels to be sure that you are not unknowingly overdoing it. Since we do not know what the safe level of consumption is for rice, just use caution and do not make it the main staple in your diet.

    Organic rice can have just as much arsenic as non-organic. Brown rice syrup also contains higher levels of arsenic since it is so concentrated. Look for this ingredient in foods since it is used as a sweetener. Rice milk should also be reconsidered if you are avoiding dairy due to the increased risk if you consume it daily. Remember those puffed rice cereals and rice cakes, too, if they are a popular food in your home. Since arsenic is a heavy metal and toxin, it should be avoided when trying to conceive. Everyone's body is different and some may be able to detox arsenic safely when they consume larger amounts of rice and rice products while others may not. Watch the serving size, too—rice can really spike blood sugar levels.

- Corn! Corn on the cob! Corn tortillas! Corn chips! Corn is beloved by many, but unfortunately it is one of the top GMO foods. If you are consuming corn, it should be organic and non-GMO. Many of us love to go out for Mexican food but along with your Tex-Mex, salsa, and margaritas, you are getting genetically modified corn chips unless otherwise stated. Please be aware of GMO corn, especially when you are trying to conceive.

- Amaranth, an ancient food staple, is not truly a grain, but often eaten like one. Nutritionally it is more like a leafy green. It contains high levels of the amino acid lysine, calcium, magnesium, and iron. In fact, with four times the amount of calcium and twice the amount of iron and magnesium than wheat, amaranth is a nutritious option. It can be cooked like other grains, or in the skillet to give it a nutty flavor. It is also sometimes put in granola or cereal.

- Buckwheat is another food thought to be a grain, but it actually is a fruit seed, gluten-free and rich in magnesium. It contains phytonutrients, which help prevent disease. It is a good protein and contains all eight essential fatty acids. Diets including buckwheat have been shown to lower the risk of developing high blood pressure and high cholesterol. Canadian researchers have also found it helps manage diabetes. Before preparing, it should be rinsed. You can also find buckwheat flour and substitute in most recipes, for example to make buckwheat muffins or pancakes.

- Millet, another gluten-free option, contains copper, manganese, phosphorus, and magnesium. It also has heart-protective properties, helps control blood sugar, and prevents gallstones. Millet originated in Africa and was used for unleavened bread. It should always be washed before cooking, and has a rice-like consistency when boiled. Millet can be eaten as porridge, added to muffins and breads, or eaten as a substitute for rice or potatoes.

- Beans are another great food. They contain a lot of fiber, iron, and folic acid. You can eat beans with a variety of dishes, as a side dish or in soups. These include garbanzo, black, pinto, kidney, cannelloni, or whatever your favorite happens to be.

- Lentils, like beans, are very high in iron, folic acid. They are great to add to soups, as a side dish, or as a lentil salad mixed with other vegetables. There are red lentils, black beluga, French green, puy, and many more varieties. They are quick, filling, and easy to prepare.

Dairy

Dairy has a place in some people's diets, while others run from it for various reasons. There are many different nutritional theories supporting or discouraging the intake of dairy as well. Some are lactose intolerant, allergic, or do not believe it should be consumed past infancy. Some people can tolerate raw dairy, but not pasteurized dairy. Each person is an individual and should go with their gut reaction—in this case, literally. How does it affect your gut? Can you tolerate butter and cheese, but not milk? Does all dairy make you gassy or have run to the restroom? Some cheeses are made with an entirely different process in the U.S. as compared to cheeses made in Europe. Some people go abroad and do fine with the dairy of other countries, but when they come home they cannot tolerate it. Cheeses made from goat or sheep's milk are easier on the stomach than those made from cow's milk.

If you do choose to consume dairy, organic is best. Be sure it does not contain rGBH (Recombinant Bovine Growth Hormone) which are banned in Europe and Australia. This hormone has been linked to cancer, and it has been shown that milk with rGBH has a lower the nutritional value than milk that is not contaminated with this growth hormone. A lot of milk is over-pasteurized as well, so finding one that has minimal processing is better for you.

You've probably heard the saying "Butter makes it better." It most certainly does! Butter can be enjoyed thoroughly when trying to conceive. New research indicates it is not the cause of cholesterol as once thought. Our ancestors thrived on the fat of butter and were much more fertile than we are today, so butter your veggies, toast, or whatever you like! Finding organic butter and butter from grass-fed cows is best. Ghee—a form of clarified butter that needs no refrigeration—is also a great option to cook with. It lasts for years, is rich in vitamins A, D, and E, and has anti-cancer and anti-inflammatory properties. When it comes to baking and cooking with butter, one of the biggest benefits is that it does not break down when heated, like other oils do, so there are fewer free radicals. In addition, most people who are lactose intolerant or avoiding casein can eat butter with no reaction. If you have not tried it, go for it since butter has such a high nutritional value.

When trying to conceive, dairy can be a good thing for the diet, as long as you can tolerate it due to the fat content. Contrary to what we learned in years past, we do need fat. For some people, it may be a good idea to avoid dairy when trying to conceive, since in Chinese medicine dairy is thought to cause stagnation or "clog" the blood. You can add it back into your diet once you are pregnant. This doesn't need to be absolute. For example, you may just need to avoid milk, cheese, and yogurt, but can still use butter or ghee. If you are wondering what to do, talk to someone who specializes in Chinese medicine and find out their point of view on dairy. All nutritionists and doctors are not created equal and will have various opinions.

If you decide to consume dairy, make sure it is organic and non-rGBH, since this is the healthiest kind.

Cooked Versus Raw Food

According to Chinese medicine, when you are trying to conceive it is best to have warm foods and a warm belly. Try preparing your foods cooked or blanched. Even sautéed pineapple is a great treat around the time of ovulation! During the summer, you're more likely to be eating raw, so trying cutting back on raw foods and meals consciously. If you still prefer a fresh green salad, go for it and see if your body agrees with that. If you are not successful at conceiving after a few months, then follow the Chinese medicine theory and switch to cooked greens and foods.

There are many dietary theories out there. No single one is correct or will work for everyone. You have to see what works for you. The key is to eat healthy, unprocessed, organic, and non-GMO. That is one way of eating to prepare for conception that most everyone can agree on.

Fertility and Pregnancy Supplements

Along with a healthy diet, most OB-GYNs and midwifes will recommend a prenatal supplement. Some are by prescription and others are available over the counter. Eating a well-balanced diet is the most important thing, but vitamins give an extra boost to your body. Because the soil today is less nutrient-rich because of the overuse of pesticides, vitamins bridge the gap between what you are getting from your food and what you need for optimal nutrition. Prenatal vitamins are especially key if you are not able to always eat organic food. While eating organic is the best option, it is not available in all areas and it can be too costly for many.

There are so many prenatal vitamins on the market that it is difficult to know which is the safest and best for our bodies. Generally speaking, we want one free of allergens, artificial colors, preservatives, and fillers. Organic is best. I would also avoid one with soy or that includes mysterious ingredients in the product's ingredient list.

Most women start taking prenatal vitamins for at least three months prior to getting pregnant, along with folate. Because folate is of the utmost importance, it is important to know that the supplements found in many grocery and drug stores are not sufficient. I use Folate 1,000 mcg by Pure Encapsulations, which has the proper type of folate (Methylfolate). According to a study, Human Genome Project this form is better because it is bio-available and reduces anemia risk.[9] "About 40% to 60% of the population has genetic polymorphisms that impair the conversion of supplemental folic acid to its active form, l-methylfolate."[10]

Women taking it had higher hemoglobin levels during the second trimester and at delivery. Having higher levels prevents iron deficiency and anemia. Klaire Labs also makes the proper form of folate. Check with your doctor to see what dosage you should be taking in addition to your multivitamin. Vitamin D is also important to keep in mind since it helps prevent fibroids according to Dr. Oz.[11] "Pregnant women with insufficient levels of vitamin D may be at increased risk of gestational diabetes, preeclampsia, and having infants small for their gestational age."[12] Make sure you are getting enough Vitamin D or just sit in the sun without sunscreen for 10-15 minutes and get Vitamin D naturally.

A good fish oil supplement (tested for toxins of course) is essential. Green Pasture makes great options, as well as Carlson. Some women also need a little extra calcium and magnesium, sometimes with added vitamin D. If you choose, you can also take evening primrose oil, maca, and royal jelly, which are all thought to help boost fertility. Coenzyme Q10 (CoQ10) is often recommended, since CoQ10 declines as you age and supports many vital functions throughout the body. CoQ10 is found in organ meats and some seafood, but is hard to obtain solely from food.

Check with your physician before starting a supplementation program, especially if you take medications regularly. Depending on your health and diet, you may need more or fewer supplements. Speak to a professional to make sure you are getting the proper amounts—while many of us can benefit from supplementation, more is not necessarily better. Do not forget to have your husband check his vitamin routine with his doctor as well. He will most likely need a multi-vitamin, fish oil or flax for the omega fats, and perhaps a vitamin E and D. You both may also need to add enzymes to your diet to help you properly break down food. These are available from Klaire Labs, Young Living, and other companies. Having a good probiotic is also recommended for both of you. I really love the probiotic Life 5 by Young Living.

Favorite Fertility Supplements

Below is a list of my favorite supplements. There are other brands out there that are good and organic. Read the ingredients and consult a health care professional who knows what your body needs.

Garden of Life Kind Organics Prenatal
Prothera Prenatal Formula
Garden of Life Kind Organic Men's Multi
Prothera VitaPrime Capsule Multi (for Men)
Methylfolate/Folate 1000 (Pure Encapsulations, Klaire Labs)
Vitamin D (Carlson, Designs for Health)
Calcium, Magnesium, Vitamin D blend
Fish Oil/Cod Liver Oil (Green Pastures, Carlson)
Evening Primrose Oil (Barleans Organic)
Maca (Navitas Naturals, Whole World Botanicals Organic)
Royal Jelly (Y.S. Eco Bee Farms)
CoQ10
Probiotic (Young Living Life 5)
Vitamin E (Carlson E Gems Elite)

Iron

It is also essential to get enough iron in your diet. Low iron can lead to anemia, and make you tired and sluggish. Note that drinking tea with a meal will limit iron absorption. Caffeine also interferes with iron absorption. It is best to eat a food higher in vitamin C with your iron-containing food for maximum absorption. Eating broccoli, oranges, grapefruit, green peppers, cabbage, or strawberries with iron-rich foods is another good option for maximum absorption.

Iron-rich Fertility Favorites

Liver from Organic Chicken or Beef
Red Meat such as Bison, Venison, or Beef

Caviar
Egg Yolks
Sesame Butter/Tahini
Clams/Oysters/Mussels
Sardines
Cocoa Powder
Sundried Tomatoes
Sunflower Seeds
Pumpkin Seeds
Thyme, Parsley
Spinach, Swiss Chard
Broccoli
Beans (Lentils, Chickpeas, Kidney, Black, Pinto, Butter, Peas or Haricot)
Curry Powder
Nuts (Almonds, Cashews, Brazil Nuts, Walnuts)
Sulfite-free Dried Apricots
Quinoa

If you cook in a cast iron pan you will naturally add iron to your food! Cast iron is also one of the safest cookware options out there.

Stay Hydrated

Water is so essential that it surprises me how often people overlook the need for proper hydration. Most are not drinking enough water, drinking soda or caffeinated beverages instead. Water is essential for the body to function properly. Clean, filtered water is even more important. Having a water filter in your home is ideal. You can easily mount one on your sink with the help of a plumber or use a filtered pitcher. Having an adequate amount of water in your body will help your cervical mucus and keep the body hydrated.

Drinking water from glass bottles is much better than from plastic bottles, as the bottles leach chemicals into the water. There are glass bottles (Lifefactory produces a good one) that can be reused so you can take your filtered water from home anywhere. There are also stainless steel options as well from companies like Kleen Kanteen. Just be sure they are in top shape with no scratches or dents. If you are out and need to purchase a beverage, opt for a glass bottle for whatever you are buying. Hopefully you are choosing tea or an apple cider vinegar drink. This is important: No sports drinks, sodas, or drinks high in carbs and sugar! There are so many options on the market for beverages it can be overwhelming when trying to choose. The majority of them contain a very high amount of sugar, carbs, and artificial ingredients. Believe it or not, sports drinks can have toxic chemicals like Brominated vegetable oil which is actually also patented as a flame retardant.[13] It is in your best interest to choose something simple when you are buying something on the go like organic tea or water. Read the ingredients, and if it does not sound natural, do not buy it.

Many people love coffee, but it dehydrates you, so it is best to avoid coffee when trying to conceive. For some people, coffee can cause a racing heart, hyperactivity, aggression, and other symptoms due to its caffeine content. If you do drink it, take careful note on how it affects you and see if it is something you should eliminate from your diet. If you must have it, buy organic, since coffee contains the highest amount of pesticides compared to other crops.[14] The other crops just as high in pesticides are tobacco and cotton.[15] "More than 1000 chemicals have been identified in roasted coffee, many of which are produced by roasting." Now if that doesn't make you want to buy organic coffee I do not know how else to convince you!

If you can choose decaffeinated, look for Swiss water processed decaf, which uses no chemicals in the decaffeination process.

There are also other newer beverage options like water kefir, kefir, and kombucha. These can be healthy, delicious, and aid in the digestive process, but be sure to read ingredients and sugar content for the best options.

Some women swear by organic red raspberry leaf tea to prepare and tone the uterus. If you like it, enjoy! You can drink it throughout pregnancy hot or cold. It should also be noted that when you are making teas at home, you should consider using organic loose leaf as opposed to tea bags. The paper the tea is contained in may not be the best for your health and leach toxins when brewed in hot water. You can find all you need to make organic loose leaf teas of all types at Mountain Rose Herbs. They have a pregnancy tea called Fecundi as well as a Nurse-Me Rhyme tea to help with breast milk production once your baby arrives.

CHAPTER FOUR: THE MOMMY MINDSET

You truly want to be a parent! But, did you know that negative emotions can affect your ability to conceive? Now that you had your body evaluated, it is time to take a look at other aspects of your health. Having a positive attitude and knowing that an amazing miracle is taking place inside of your belly will hopefully make you better able to manage any pregnancy ache, pain, or inconvenience. This is important because your baby can feel your negative emotions! Focusing on the negative can affect the way you feel physically and emotionally, and also drain your energy.

If you are stressed, confused, or not getting enough rest, it is important to ask yourself: *Do I have unresolved issues that I need to explore?* Maybe you are nervous about this journey to parenthood and are unsure if now is the right time. Whatever you are feeling, it is most likely normal, but, if need be, seek the advice of a professional. This chapter all boils down to having the right attitude. Before beginning your journey to parenthood, take a breath. Make sure you truly understand what a special and amazing time pregnancy can be. Think about it: You are creating (or about to create) a life—a beautiful, new life that will grow inside of you. Nurture this life with the right nutrition and by taking great care of you. When you truly take the time to listen and care for your body, rest when you need to, and get adequate sleep, pregnancy can be a joyous experience!

Staying Positive During Your Pregnancy

Begin by thinking of your pregnancy as a 40-41-week marathon that you go through with strength, pride, perseverance, gratitude, stamina, energy, joy, bliss, happiness, love, and peace! If you can set yourself up with this mindset, then you will be a great success. Mind over matter, or body, if you like, makes such a huge impact.

First pregnancies can be scary for some women. You do not know what to expect or how you are supposed to feel. There are many moments when you wonder if the things that are happening to your body are normal. Pregnancy can definitely be a physically and mentally grueling process, but there are natural things you can do to relieve almost any issue during pregnancy. Granted, you may have to put up with some nausea and sleepiness in the first trimester. You might also have preexisting medical conditions, which could make your pregnancy harder than it typically is for the average woman. I suggest that you push through with gratitude and perseverance, knowing that you can do this! You *can* have a healthy pregnancy.

Talking to friends or an online support group can be helpful as long as the conversation doesn't turn negative. Seek out those with a similar mindset. Talk to your doctor, midwife, or doula when needed. They will know how best to help you and can remind you that having a baby is a natural process to be enjoyed and cherished. Remember: Attitude is everything. Staying positive while pregnant even though you may have a challenging pregnancy can make all the difference. When you improve your overall mindset, you will most likely notice that your physical ailments are less worrisome.

Be grateful for the life you are creating. This perspective can make many things seem less stressful. Lorraine Miller's *From Gratitude to Bliss: A Journey in Health and Happiness* is a gratitude journal that can help you log what you have to be grateful for on a daily basis. She created it to help women incorporate daily gratitude into their lives. We sometimes take for granted what we have and lust for more. Being grateful every day puts us in a positive mindset and reduces stress—both are ingredients for an enjoyable pregnancy! Do what you can to incorporate a daily gratitude practice into your life and see how it makes a difference for you.

Seeking Help

If you have discomfort, treat it naturally if possible. From acupuncturists to herbalists, chiropractors to cranial sacral practitioners, yoga masters to therapists, Reiki masters to hypnotherapists, there are many specialists who will be happy to help you during your pregnancy. For example, if you have deep fears about pregnancy, a hypnotherapist can be especially helpful for some. For others, this may be a good time to take up meditation or another restorative practice. The idea is to find something that helps you relax and feel good about the journey you are about to embark on. Focusing your mind and body on becoming a parent in a natural, healthy way can help and—with as little stress as possible—can help the reproductive process go easier.

If faith is important to you, no matter what your religion, prayer has been known to bring about all sorts of miracles. Prayer *can* work wonders! Having faith and a deep belief in a higher power and letting your true desire be known (about wanting to become a parent) may be the extra touch needed to create a new life inside of you. People trying to conceive have had success being part of a prayer chain or a prayer circle for healing. When nothing else works scientifically, prayer is what a lot of people believe brings about their babies.

Managing Stress

Part of your mental health check in includes looking at your stress levels and at how stress affects you. It has such a huge effect on our health, whether we realize it or not. Stress can negatively affect fertility, too. If you need to make changes in your life, steps to de-stress can be taken one day at a time, one week at a time, or at whatever pace feels right to you.

The way the majority of people live their lives today does not create a healthy environment for conception. We are overworked, overscheduled, overcommitted, and overstressed. This kind of stress leads to many health problems, some of which we are not aware of until we have a major problem in our body. That nagging headache, inability to sleep, or tension in the shoulders, these can all be signs of stress. Stress can affect hormonal levels like causing cortisol and epinephrine levels to skyrocket. If you are continually run-down, tired, and stressed out, how is that going to affect conceiving? If you do become pregnant, how will that affect the baby and pregnancy?

Take a look at your current employment situation: maybe make a career change or cut down the number of hours you work. The long hours some of us work are grueling. Many times we rise early, go to work, come home, and go to sleep without having a moment to ourselves. We squeeze meals in between working hours or rush through them, gobbling down unhealthy options. This is not how life is meant to be. Remember the saying, *All work and no play*? If you are reading this and you see yourself at this extreme, take a deep breath and relax. You can and should make a change for the sake of yourself and your future baby, even if that means earning less income. Taking the necessary steps to streamline your overworked mind and body will give you a greater chance at becoming pregnant. You need to focus on becoming a parent and making as many healthy choices as possible!

How about your social life? Do you spend many late nights out with friends? Maybe you are someone who says yes to every social event you are presented with, no matter how busy you are. Pre-baby is an exciting time, when many of your friends are getting engaged, getting married, celebrating big birthdays, buying homes, taking vacations, and having parties just to have a party. As fun as it is to be a part of joyous occasions, if being the social butterfly and attending all the events you are invited to stresses you out, you can pass! If you truly want to become a parent, take a step back and listen to how your body responds to your lifestyle.

While social commitments may not be stressful in the moment, they can be stressful on the body if they encourage you to eat poorly, drink alcohol, and get little sleep. Politely decline invitations, and let your close friends know you are trying to conceive and do not want to over-schedule your social life. Spend your evenings and weekends relaxing and taking care of your body and emotional well-being with a few social outings sprinkled in here and there.

Eating before a party helps you make wise choices. Also, when you do dine out, you have options—you can have your cake and eat it too! The importance of refraining from alcohol and other substances while you are pregnant should go without saying. In case you were wondering, these activities are no-no's as early as three months prior to conception, if you are trying to create the healthiest eggs and sperm. As you prepare for the conception that your partner and you so deeply desire, having this kind of lifestyle should become your first priority.

Relationships

Relationships can also be a form of stress. Hopefully the relationship you have with your partner is in the right place to begin with before you conceive. If it needs a fine-tuning, seek out a counselor or group therapy class. Whatever works for you in order to strengthen your relationship. The main point is to ensure you both are on the same page as far as pregnancy and parenting. This is a major game-changer in some relationships, and unfortunately not all couples weather the storm of parenting well. The pregnancy may be blissful, but once it is time to change dirty diapers and clean soiled laundry in addition to all of the other changes around a home with a new baby, arguments and resentments can ensue.

Having a strong foundation in your relationship—one that is free of stress—can make all the difference prior to pregnancy. Answering those questions that come up during the early days of parenthood will make situations less difficult to deal with once baby is already here. Who does the nighttime duty? Who changes the diapers? Who cooks and cleans, or shops? Are all of the duties shared? Maybe you set aside a budget to have someone help with these duties, or ask family or friends to help out. Making life easier and less stressful will give everyone some relief and extra time to enjoy the new bundle of joy.

Personal relationships can also wear you down and stress you out. These can be with friends, family, or with co-workers. Whatever the case, relationships should be productive, lift your spirits, and be a positive influence. If a relationship no longer serves you, there are a few options. First, you can limit the time you spend with people who are negative or suck the energy out of you. Second, you can also decline invitations to meet with them. Be honest and tell them that your ideas, interests, and lives are going in different directions and you have other commitments! There is no need to be rude, but you can politely get your point across and keep your stress level down. Who wants to spend time with people they don't enjoy or people who do not share the same beliefs and lifestyle?

For relationships you cannot avoid, such as family or co-workers, my best advice is to remain calm and make small shifts to keep stress levels low. If a work situation is really bad, it may be time for a job change or at least a talk with your boss. If you have plans to spend time with someone who really bothers you, meditate before seeing them. Meditation is one way to protect yourself from other people's negative energy. Remember: Stress is not good for conception or baby. So breathe, count to ten, diffuse or wear essential oils, or do whatever else works for you. Repeat when necessary!

Importance of Sleep

Sleep is another factor that dramatically affects a pregnancy. Many underestimate the need for rest. Our ability to conceive is affected by the amount of sleep we get. Sleep deprivation can increase the risk of miscarriage or lead to other problems during pregnancy as well. The forming of eggs and sperms happens around the clock, but our bodies need the proper amount of sleep to function. Some people feel they need less while others cannot function unless they have seven or eight hours of sleep, or more. We really need at least seven to nine hours in order for our bodies to go through an adequate sleep cycle, no matter our age.

Lack of sleep can contribute to many health problems. We need sleep in order to repair our bodies and cells and to fight off infections and disease, and healing happens while we sleep. According to Dr. Rubin Naiman, PhD, sleep specialist, and clinical assistant professor of the University Arizona's Center for Integrative Medicine, one in four men and one in nine women suffer from a sleep disorder. Seventy million people in the United States suffer from insomnia.[16] Inadequate amounts of sleep can lead to obesity, diabetes, insulin resistance, cancer, arthritis, mood disorders, and infection. Our circadian rhythms—the body clock that tells us when to sleep—can be thrown off balance. We should be sleeping at night when it is dark. If your circadian rhythm is off, so too is the rest of your system.

Sleep deprivation can hurt both partners' ability to reproduce. It affects hormone levels, often increasing levels of the stress hormone cortisol. If women do not get enough sleep, they may not produce adequate levels of the hormone leptin, a hormone which is associated with ovulation. This can cause irregular menstrual cycles and affect your fertility. Men who do not get enough sleep can suffer from lower sperm counts and low testosterone levels. No man wants to hear that! Say goodbye to late night movies or surfing the Internet, gentleman, and protect your sperm production.

We need to be making strong and healthy eggs and sperm. If our bodies are not in top form by getting the necessary sleep, we are bound to be less capable of producing top quality eggs and sperm. By getting the deepest sleep in the first part of the night, experiencing the dreaming stage during the latter third of the night—which includes the deep REM sleep that is needed—our bodies heal emotionally and physically. If you are on anti-depressants, they will suppress your dreaming or REM sleep, which is a critical part of the sleep cycle. If we do not get seven to nine hours of sleep, our metabolism kicks into overdrive and we are hungrier and more prone to overeating when we awake.

In addition, the hours before midnight are the most restorative hours for the body to heal and regenerate. Every hour of sleeping before midnight is thought to be worth two hours. This is especially important once you have children. Children need these restorative hours even more so than we do as adults, so it is helpful to instill an early bedtime for them, too.

By getting more sleep, you are being "green" by having the lights, TV, and computer off. Most likely you are under a blanket, so the heat is turned down a bit during the winter months. The need to stay up late to "get things done" or to relax in front of the TV should be rethought. Relaxing or resting is not the same as sleeping. Lack of sleep puts stress on the body and mind. It can cause unclear thinking or the inability to focus. In fact, driving after too little sleep can be as dangerous as driving under the influence of alcohol.

There are steps you can take to help you fall asleep easier, but don't let these stress you out so you can't sleep! According to Dr. Naiman, sleeping pills are not the solution and may increase cancer risk more than smoking! A low carb, sugar free diet is best. Avoiding alcohol and caffeine should also help you sleep better. You should not have a light on in the room—make it as dark as possible. You can even wear blue blocker glasses or a sleeping mask to block out light. Add room-darkening shades to your room to prevent light from coming in from the windows. One of the most important steps is to limit screen time before bed. Being on the computer or watching television before bed can severely affect your ability to fall and stay asleep. Instead, meditation, yoga, or breathing exercises can quiet your mind and body much better.

Another diet-sleep tip is to stay away from foods high in the amino acid tyrosine to help you fall asleep easier. If you suffer from insomnia, avoid these high-tyrosine foods: fermented meats and cheeses, beer and wine, certain dairy and soy products, and seeds. While some of these foods are good for conception and should be part of a balanced diet, some—like the fermented meats and dairy—should be eaten sparingly, because they may not agree with your body when it comes time to go to sleep. If you still want to eat them, eliminate them from your dinner meal. If that does not work, you may need to try avoiding them at lunchtime as well. See what works for you in order to get a full night sleep.

FOODS TO AVOID FOR A RESTFUL SLEEP

Fermented meats, like pepperoni
Fermented cheeses, like cheddar
Avocados
Beer
Wine
Chicken
Soy products
Fish
Turkey
Peanuts
Almonds
Bananas
Lima beans
Sesame
Pumpkin seeds
Yogurt
Cottage cheese
Milk

Your body needs melatonin in order to sleep. As we age, the melatonin produced by the body declines. Rather than taking a supplement, which is not melatonin's natural form, try adding foods rich in melatonin to your diet at dinner or before bedtime. These foods include pineapples, oranges, raspberries, oats and oatmeal, sweet corn, rice, tomatoes, a tablespoon of flax seeds, walnuts, orange bell peppers, a teaspoon of fenugreek or mustard seed, and goji or lyceum berries. According to research, the best food source for melatonin production is cherries, which should be eaten an hour before bed.[17] Try tart cherry juice, which contains less sugar and more melatonin. Organic and non-GMO is best for all of these foods, except for pineapples, which contain few pesticides. If you are watching your blood sugar levels, it is best to have these after dinner rather than right before bed. This protects you from waking up with elevated blood sugar.

FOODS TO PROMOTE SLEEP CONTAINING MELATONIN

Cherries, tart cherry juice (best option)
Pineapples
Oranges
Raspberries
Oats or oatmeal
Non-GMO sweet corn
Non-GMO Rice
Tomatoes
Flax seeds (tablespoon)
Walnuts
Orange bell peppers
Fenugreek (teaspoon)
Mustard seed
Goji berries
Lyceum berries

When you add more sleep to your routine, you will feel refreshed and ready to go in the morning. The sperm and egg quality and necessary hormones will be given the best chance by getting a restful night's sleep. You will also have more energy for sex, which should make conceiving more fun, rather than a chore. In addition, getting an adequate amount of sleep can help the body heal from injuries and illness at a faster rate. It can also help regulate gestational diabetes fasting numbers, too.

However you choose to clear your mind, change your attitude, and remove stress from your life is up to you. Do not feel the need to try everything—that can stress you out, too. Be grateful every day, smile, and stay positive. Make a plan and stick to it. Set a clear time for bed every night and follow through with it. After a few weeks of following a routine, eliminating stress, and getting adequate sleep you will feel a difference and be on the road to bliss!

CHAPTER FIVE: DETOX YOUR BEAUTY, CLEANING AND HOUSEHOLD

Cosmetics are a necessity for some women. If this is you, now is the time to clean out your makeup bag and medicine cabinet! The chemicals found in the majority of beauty products are toxic to you and your eggs. Most women never think about the ingredients that are in their makeup or beauty products. Use your best judgment and limit exposure to chemicals prior to and during pregnancy. You are what you eat, but you are also what you put on your skin and what you breathe.

The skin is the largest organ in the body, and it absorbs whatever chemicals you put on it. Many makeups contain harsh and toxic ingredients. Women simply put on lipstick without a thought, unknowingly—in many cases—applying lead to their lips. Creams and moisturizers, also absorbed into the skin, can also affect our health. Often, they contain parabens (which are banned in other countries) and polyethylene glycols (PEGs). Some of these ingredients, like parabens, are endocrine disruptors, which affect hormones and overall health. Phthalates are linked to birth defects as well.

When putting on makeup, you also breathe in small particles from powders, blushes, and eye shadows. These particles can contain large amounts of lead and other heavy metals such as arsenic, selenium, and mercury—none of which you want to get into your lungs. This includes some mineral makeups, which sound safe since minerals come from the earth even though they are made from unsafe ingredients.

Propylene glycol is another ingredient to watch out for, as are any other products with chemicals that include the word "glycol" for that matter. "Depending on manufacturing processes, PEGs can be contaminated with measurable amounts of ethylene oxide and 1,4-dioxane. The International Agency for Research on Cancer classifies ethylene oxide as a known human carcinogen and 1,4-dioxane as a possible human carcinogen."[18]

There are no regulations on what companies can put in makeup, but strides are being made by the Campaign for Safe Cosmetics to get companies to make safer, non-toxic products that don't harm us or our developing babies.[19] If what we put on our skin is toxic, it is a danger and can affect us when trying to conceive whether we know it or not. Hormones play a vital role in our conceiving, and using products that alter their levels is a great cause of concern. There are safer options available made without fragrances or toxic chemicals. We need to be more aware of them and take extra caution in choosing them when we are thinking about conceiving. Don't be fooled by the words "natural" or "eco-friendly" because that does not mean they contain totally safe ingredients. These are terms used in marketing products and have no bearing on what is actually in the product, since there are no regulations.

Non Toxic Makeup Favorites

100% Pure
Devita
Gabriel Cosmetics
Zulu Cosmetics
Honeybee Gardens
Tata Harper
Young Living Lip Balm
Badger Sunscreen & bug repellant
www.spiritbeautylounge.com

Besides, when you are pregnant you are glowing from the inside out and should really embrace this pregnancy beauty.

Once in a while, try going with less makeup or without any and embrace your true beauty. You will have less time to spend in the mirror once your baby arrives anyway.

There are dangerous ingredients used in the beauty industry. There are things you may not be aware of that you do or put on your body on a daily, weekly or monthly basis that expose you to dangerous toxins.

- Fragrances are a big offender. They are made in a lab full of synthetic chemicals, which are not found in nature. Some are used in makeups and lotions, while others are found in typical perfumes. They contain phthalates and other harsh chemicals, and should really be avoided. Many people can't walk past a makeup or perfume counter without becoming nauseated or getting a headache. They are the so called "canaries in the coal mine." Their bodies are letting them know these products are not good for them. If you must use a fragrance, try using essential oils of good quality that are therapeutic grade like Young Living's Essential Oils. There are also a number of non-toxic perfumes coming on the market. You just need to look a little harder to find them. Be sure to read the ingredients in your makeup as well to avoid fragrance, unless it is from an essential oil.
- Baby powder and similar powder products contain *talc*—which many of us think is safe. "Commonly found in baby powders, face powders, body powders. Talc is a known carcinogen and is a major cause of ovarian cancer. It can be harmful if inhaled as it can lodge in the lungs, causing respiratory disorders. Since the early 1980s, records show that several thousand infants each year have died or become seriously ill following accidental inhalation of baby powder."[20]
- Nail salons should also be avoided. The amounts of chemicals found in nail salons are enough to knock you over! They can make you ill and possibly affect your fertility, unless you find one using nontoxic polishes and removers. Their products should

be free of toluene, dibutyl phthalates, and formaldehyde. They can also be found in hairsprays. Those are the major chemicals to watch out for but unfortunately there are others not as readily tested for safety. A North Carolina study reported higher rates of miscarriage among nail salon employees. The fact that there is even a study about such a thing should raise a concern.

- Hair care is something we all must attend to. A salon that uses nontoxic products is a great goal, but not available to all. You can bring your own organic nontoxic shampoo with you to the salon and ask them to use it before you get a trim. If you do color your hair, wait at least until the second trimester when the risk of miscarriage is much less and use a natural colorant from a nontoxic salon. You are exposed to toxic chemicals just by being in the salon near others who are getting coloring, perms, straightening, or Brazilian blowouts, etc. While your exposure is much less than the employees working in the salon, you never know how much toxic exposure your own body or your unborn baby can withstand.

- Avoid spray on tans, tanning beds and skin whitening, too. The heat from tanning and the chemicals used for whitening or spray tans have not all been tested properly. Let nature do what it is intended to do, and do what you can to produce a healthy baby. Do not alter your appearance by tanning or whitening your skin through artificial means during or before pregnancy. It's best to continue being cautious after birth while breastfeeding, too. Not enough evidence on safety is known about these procedures or chemicals used. Why take a chance?

- Would you like to whiten your teeth while pregnant? Do not use the harmful over-the-counter products or anything strong from a dentist. You can do it naturally with baking soda, coconut oil, or apple cider vinegar. You would be amazed at how white your teeth can get from simply using baking soda or trying oil pulling with coconut oil.

- Wondering if you need a prescription for the bothersome pregnancy-induced acne? Think again! Accutane, Retin-A, and

Tetracycline are extremely dangerous before conception and during pregnancy. There are other drugs that may be safer, but your safest option is to maintain a healthy diet and use something more natural to halt acne. You can add essential oils, like lavender, lemon, or Frankincense, into a little organic raw coconut oil for healthy skin support. When using lemon, be sure to avoid direct sunlight after applying, because it may cause you to be more sensitive to the sun. Facials should also be avoided, unless you know the products contain safe ingredients. You can give yourself a facial with egg whites and oatmeal. The results will surprise you!

- Antiperspirants containing aluminum should be tossed in the trash! This may be a tough one for some women to change, but there is a possible link between aluminum and breast cancer, reproductive failure, and ovarian lesions in mice (according to one study).[21] The parabens and phthalates used in many antiperspirants are hazardous as well. There are safer alternatives like a Crystal stick or roll on. You can find safer options at the store if you take a little time to look.

  Honestly, if you have a clean diet then your body should not be emitting much odor in the first place. Eating pork or beef, spicy foods, dairy, and sometimes cruciferous vegetables, if not cooked enough, can contribute to more body odor. So can processed foods and junk food. Having a low carb diet can cause the body to emit odors, too. A balanced diet is essential, just be aware of what foods you eat that contribute to an odor. Many women find that when they clean up their diet, they do not even need deodorant.

- As far as hand soaps go, look for the ingredient Triclosan (in addition to other harmful ingredients). Triclosan is extremely toxic and most likely in the soap you find in public bathrooms. The best advice is to carry a sample size bottle of your own non-toxic soap and some natural non-toxic hand sanitizer, instead of polluting your body with questionable products when you are out and about. If you do not know what ingredients are in these products, you can't protect your eggs or your unborn child.

- Sunscreens and bug repellants go on our skin then absorb into our bloodstream. They sometimes are already in our makeup or sold individually. Many of these brands that claim to protect you from harm, actually contain ingredients harmful to your skin and body. Chose products carefully!

Ingredients and Chemicals to Avoid

Here is a list of ingredients to look for in your beauty-related products. You will notice that the first ingredient talc, which, many believe is safe. This will give you an idea of just how little you may know about the products you use every day.

Talc

Fragrance

Sodium laurel sulfate

Sodium Laureth

Mineral oil

Petroleum jelly or petrolatum

Parabens

DEA

MEA

TEA

DBP or Dibutyl phthalates

Triclosan (hand soaps-antibacterial)

Aluminum

Heavy metals: Lead, Mercury, Cadmium, Arsenic, Nickel

p-Phenylenediamine

DMDM Hydantoin

Diazolidinyl urea

Imidazolidinyl Urea

Methenamine

Quarternium-15

PEGs
Siloxanes (Cyclomethicone and ingredients ending in "siloxane" such as Cyclotetrasiloxane)

Differin (Adapelene)

Retin-A, Renova (Tretinoin)

Retinoic acid

Retinol

Retinyl Linoleate

Retinyl Palmitate

Tazorac and Avage (Tazarotene)
Salicylic acid

Beta hydroxy acid

BHA
Lethicin

Soy

Textured vegetable protein (TVP)
Potassium Thioglycolate (depilatory)

Calcium Thioglycolate (depilatory)

Sodium Hydroxide (minimizer)

Hydrolyzed Soy Protein (minimizer)

Sanguisorba Officinalis Root Extract (minimizer)

If this list overwhelms you, you are not alone. These ingredients and industrial chemicals, which we ingest through our skin, are found to be carcinogens, pesticides, reproductive toxins, and endocrine disruptors.

Many of the chemicals and toxic ingredients found in beauty-related products are also used in manufacturing and cleaning! Why on earth would we want these on our skin? And why would a company think it is safe to put on skin? It is truly scary what we are exposed to on a daily basis in the name of beauty! Switching out your current makeup for safer, non-toxic and organic products is one of the best investments you can make for yourself. In the long run you can teach your daughters and granddaughters to choose safe makeup. We all want to look pretty, but it should not cost us our health.

You can find safer options on the Environmental Working Group's website (www.ewg.org/skin deep) for many safer options to cosmetics that include information on every chemical in a product. This is a great resource to see how your products stack up to the safer alternatives. Also look at www.safecosmetics.org to learn more about cosmetics. Remember that while beauty is from within, if your moisturizer (or other beauty product) wreaks havoc on your hormones as it is absorbed by your skin, it is not likely to aid in a beautiful conception.

Green and Non-toxic Household Items

While your eggs and your husband's sperm are maturing inside of you, you want to protect them. This means avoiding another common consumer product—household cleaners. These contain chemicals that are truly toxic to your health, too. Who enjoys cleaning? Some people like to! Most of us have to. Since it's a fact of life for most of us, learn how to *clean green.*

Breathing in the fumes from toxic cleaners should be avoided by everyone, not just those hoping to procreate. Over the years the varieties of cleaning products claiming to be nontoxic has skyrocketed. There are many brands on the market that are safe, but many others try to "greenwash" you into believing that their products are safer than they really are. Unfortunately, the majority of products available to clean with are still highly toxic, and many have ingredients that are questionable. When you walk down the cleaning isle at the supermarket, you are bombarded with an array of scents, fragrances and chemicals not safe for anyone let alone those trying to conceive. From ammonia to bleach the list of hazards seems never-ending.

The least toxic items you can use to clean with are white grain vinegar, baking soda, lemons, salt, hydrogen peroxide, glycerin soap, beeswax, olive oil, and castile soap. While making your own cleaning recipe may seem difficult, it is easy, safe, and a lot less expensive than the pre-made toxic concoctions. You can find recipes online—and add essential oils and scents to the solutions, according to your preferences. Baking soda is my favorite to apply to grease stains, clean tubs, sinks, and just about anything! Mix with a little water to make a paste. Here are some other suggestions:

- If you have a clogged drain, try about a 1/2 to 1 cup of baking soda down the drain, followed by a cup of white vinegar. It will fizz a bit. Then add a pot of boiling water to unclog the drain.

Works in most cases! Try doing this every so often to prevent major clogs. It is much healthier than the fumes of from the drain cleaners you can purchase in the supermarket and much less than the cost of a plumber!

- Another must-have, which is great for nontoxic cleaning, is a steamer for floors or a handheld steamer. Don't use the chemical cleaners that come with some of them, they can be toxic.

- As far as laundry goes, go for detergents free of phosphates, chlorine bleach (sodium hypochlorite), and fragrances or perfumes. These are the most harmful ingredients. Also avoid any detergent with a petroleum product. A great addition to your natural laundry detergent is a cup of baking soda, since it whitens and removes odors too. If you like a fragrance, add a Young Living Essential oil such as lavender, or Purification for smelly clothes. You can also add a ball of wool to the dryer to prevent static.

- If you must dry clean some of your clothes, look for a dry cleaner who does not use Perchloroethylene (PERC). This solvent is highly toxic and should be avoided. There is risk to the workers at the dry cleaner and those who live near one. High exposure to PERC could increase the risk of developing cancer.[22] Imagine what it does to those developing eggs and sperm to those that are exposed! If you have clothes from a regular dry cleaner, the best thing to do is air them out in the garage or outside. Your exposure is hopefully minimal. Then find a dry cleaner who does not use PERC. You can find one at www.greencleanerscouncil.com.

- Also to be avoided are moths balls for storing clothes. Cedar is best to keep the moths away.

- Do not use flea and tick repellants containing DEET. They stay in clothes and are toxic to skin.

If you don't have time to make homemade cleaners, there are certain ingredients and chemicals that you should be made aware of and avoid, since they contain the harshest ingredients. Avoid oven, toilet, tub and tile cleaners; carpet and upholstery shampoo; air fresheners; dish detergents; and antibacterial cleaners. These products contain Chlorine, Formaldehyde, Triclosan (Dioxin), Phenol, Sodium Hydroxide (lye), Benzene, Toluene, Xylene, Methanol, and Ethyl benzene, (some are known carcinogens like formaldehyde and benzene) Perchloroethylene (used in dry cleaning), hydrochloric acid, and ammonia.[23]

The fact that they are easily available for purchase across the aisle from baby food is astounding! Think of the fumes you inhale or chemicals you may accidentally touch when you are using these products. The warning labels are there for a reason! Anything that could send you to the emergency room should not be in your home, EVER. Surprisingly, companies are not required to accurately label all of the ingredients found in their products, which is why avoiding them is the best idea. You do not know exactly what you are getting.

If you do not wish to make your own, you can find safer alternatives to typical cleaning products at www.ewg.org/guides/cleaners. Having a clean home is important but having it cleaned without toxins is even more essential. The products you are cleaning with will affect you now and eventually your baby!

Nontoxic Cleaning Favorites

Baking Soda
Vinegar
Peroxide
Salt
Lemons
Young Living Thieves Cleaner
Young Living Essential Oils
Earth Friendly Products
Shaklee

Toxins in Everyday Household Items

Now is the time to think about detoxing your home one household item at a time. Have you ever considered that the furniture in your home could be contributing to your allergies, asthma, or ability to conceive? Well, some of these everyday items in your home could be throwing your hormones out of balance because they are treated with flame retardants and made with other harmful chemicals like formaldehyde. Yes—I said formaldehyde again—it is a preservative in so many products.

- The first item I think of detoxing is the bed. After all, it is where most babies are created! Your everyday mattress contains many, many chemicals, which are emitted into the air each time you lay on it. You could also have dust mites or bedbugs (mistakenly brought home from a trip to an infested hotel) hiding inside your mattress. If I am grossing you out, I hope it causes you to take action. The majority of us spend most of our time in bed. During that time, you will breathe substances that affect your health. Why not choose ones that won't affect it in a negative way.

- The best choice for a mattress is an all-natural latex mattress that does not contain harmful chemicals. One made with a wool or organic cotton cover is also preferable. There are many options available now like Naturepedic, Natura, and Royal Pedic, at several price points too. A latex pillow is also your best bet, plus it deters dust mites. Some polyester pillows or feather pillows can get moist if you sweat in your sleep. If not washed or replaced frequently enough, you can have mold growing in your pillow! You can breathe a little easier knowing you made the investment in your health by choosing latex.

- Next up is the couch, sofa, or easy chair. Most of these pieces contain flame retardants, which are quite toxic. The problem is that flame retardants decompose into the air we breathe. The documentary Toxic Hot Seat[24] links flame retardants to cancer in fire fighters exposed to flame retardants as they burn. Many cushions are wrapped in toxic retardant chemicals today. If you have an older sofa or chair that has been recovered, it is likely that the cushions are made from harmful materials as well. Fortunately, a bill was passed very recently overturning the mandatory use of flame retardants on sofas. There is, however, a standing inventory of furniture still on the market containing these toxic materials. Check with the manufacturer before you buy a new piece of furniture to see if it was made with or without flame retardants. Buying a used sofa may seem like a greener thing to do, but if you are trying to conceive and avoid chemicals, don't. Also, beware of children's carseats treated with flame retardants. Many products made of fabric have a tag with the code CA 117 which means it has flame retardants. I have found many baby products from baby swings to high chair covers containing a tag with this code. The soft cushions and fabric have been treated, avoid them!

Leather is also a safer option as the dust mites aren't in the fabric and hopefully the toxins are sealed beneath the leather. At least that is what I keep telling myself as I sit on my leather sofa. It is easier to clean once kids or pets spill or slobber on it!

- Carpeting is a big contributor to household allergens. The majority of carpet is treated with a stain repellent, and it accumulates dust mites. The older the carpet, the more toxins likely. They are in the carpet padding as well. Your best option is to have a home with hardwood floors, which can be easily cleaned and which eliminate the dust mite concern. If you must have carpeting, choose a natural wool option or an area rug that can be cleaned. Depending on your style and where you live, you may also like the option of ceramic tile floors. They are an easy to clean option that can be complemented with beautiful area rugs. Compared to wood, they are also very durable and can withstand years of kids and pets running over them.

- Also look at your window coverings. Are they beautiful fabric draperies that possibly contain a flame retardant or wrinkle-free fabric treatment? If so, they too can harbor dust mites and toxic chemicals. They are costly to replace and may not need replacing right away, but when it is time, a safer option is wood blinds or curtains that are made from a safer fabric—one that is not treated with chemicals. Please avoid any cheap plastic blinds or shades, since they are most likely made of vinyl or PVC plastic. When these are in your windows and the sun hits them, the heat causes them to off-gas into your home. This affects the air quality and you begin breathing in toxins. If you have these now and cannot afford to replace them, an air purifier can help as well as the house plants mentioned to clean the air.

- Do you have an old shower curtain? Get rid of your vinyl shower curtain or your vinyl bath mat, which is full of chemicals/ phthalates that will disrupt your endocrine system. Phthalates can lower sperm counts and have been linked to endometriosis, too. A better option is one made from cloth. It works just as well without the off-gassing or plastic smell!

- Have you eliminated plastic bottles for drinking water? If so, good for you and for "greening" your life! The toxins from the plastic can leach into the water. They are also not good for the environment. Reusable glass water bottles are the safest option, when filled with filtered water. A must have in our home is filtered water for drinking and for the shower or bath. If you are not able to put in a whole house water filtration system, the next best option is a faucet mounted on the sink for drinking. It can be easily installed by a plumber, and the cost is low compared to an entire house system.

- The second must is a filtered showerhead. This can eliminate most major hazards found in water. You can buy one online and install it yourself. Aquasauna makes an easy to install showerhead that needs changing about every six months. It removes about 90 percent of chlorine and synthetic chemicals. Your skin is your largest organ, so be sure that the water you wash with is clean and non-toxic.

- If you don't have a whole-house water filtration system, you can buy a Rainshower de-chlorinator. These are perfect if you are bathing kids or enjoying a relaxing bath yourself. You can also just turn on the shower to fill up the bathtub if you have a filtered showerhead. It takes a little longer, but still does the job.

Healthy House Plants to Clean the Air

Aloe

Spider Plant

Peace Lily (Spathiphyllum)

Dracaena

Chrysanthemum

Bamboo Palm

Golden Pothos (Epipremnum aureum)

English Ivy

Chinese Evergreen

Areca Palm

Rubber Plant (Ficus elastica)

Boston Fern

Kitchen Items

Next are cooking items! Now that you (hopefully) have your diet in check before pregnancy, take a look at what you are cooking your food in on a daily basis. Remember the years of cooking with Teflon? If you missed the memo, remove all Teflon and non-stick cookware from your home. Tests showing that the chemicals emitted from the cookware were high enough to kill a bird! We may not be as small as birds but our eggs, sperm, and embryos are even smaller.

- The safest options for cooking are cast iron, glass, and enamel cookware. Some believe stainless is safe, but if it is scratched, nickel can leach into the food and then to our bodies. Cast iron has been used for ages, and it is the least expensive to find. Although it is heavy, it lasts for years and cooking with it gives your body a healthy dose of iron (in the food) as a bonus. Glass is very safe, but is easily broken. If you have a gas stovetop and drop it on the metal stove eyes, it makes for a messy, hazardous clean-up. Glass is excellent for baking and storing food, though. My favorite cookware by far is enamel cookware. It comes in an array of colors, which make your kitchen and cooking experience more beautiful. A wonderful, long-lasting brand is Le Creuset. You can find them on sale or at outlet malls at great prices. This cookware is safe and lasts for years and years.
- If you do a lot of baking, invest in stainless steel cupcake tins or use non-toxic liners, stainless cookie sheets, and other baking items. Glass bakeware is good for breads, pies and sheet cakes. The options for safe baking are few since the market is riddled with non-stick cookware. Avoid silicone for now. It has not been on the market very long, and some research indicates that it may not be safe when heated. It also contains fillers, which may get into food while cooking. It is not worth taking a chance on. The silicone utensils are somewhat safe, just do not cook or bake in items made from silicone.
- Also avoid cling wrap or plastic wrap to cover or store food. Better choices for food storage are glass containers, reusable toxin-free bags, or parchment paper.
- What are you drinking your beverages in? Hopefully, you are drinking from glass and not plastic. What are you serving your food on? Make sure it is dinnerware and china that is free from

lead paint—which is the case for most china and dinnerware on the market today. Some decorations on older china contain lead paint, which can get on your food. Check your favorite heirloom tea set, teacups and serving platters for any decorations that could contain lead paint. If so, use these items for decoration, not for serving food. If you find a lot of items, don't let the list become overwhelming. Tackle one project at a time!

• If you have plastic storage containers or other gadgets made of plastic, be careful how you use them. Plastics are good for storing something other than food, such as craft supplies or tools. If your plastic kitchen items are BPA free, that does not mean they are safe. New research shows the chemicals used in making the plastics can be just as hazardous. I know toddlers throw plates at times, so plastic is a good option to avoid breakage. Just be sure the food is cool if using plastic. Glass is best to store your food in whether for lunch or in the refrigerator. Stainless steel is another option, but be sure that it has no scratches and is in good condition. There are companies that make wood and bamboo dishes, which are a great eco-friendly option.

• When it comes to utensils, think about what you are using to feed your family and future children. Plastic utensils are Ok once in a while at a picnic, but for everyday use stainless steel is a really good option. You may want to rethink plastic as well when it's time to feed your new baby. They make plenty of options out of stainless steel, wood, or bamboo for baby and toddler spoons and forks when you start feeding baby first foods. An even better option is sterling silver. You may be saying "my baby was not born with a silver spoon in his mouth". It may not be in the budget. There is some interesting history behind why sterling silver can be a beneficial option. For centuries, the kings and queens used sterling silver while the peasants used earthenware and other metals to eat their food. There was a big difference in their health. The silver from the utensils wears away somewhat with use and your body reaps the benefits of the silver. Colloidal Silver has been used for decades for health care and is still used today. It is germicidal, wipes out disease causing bacteria, viruses, molds, parasites and fungi. It is even thought to be a natural antibiotic. Buying just one silver spoon and fork for your baby or each member of your household may have more benefits than just using fancy silverware at dinner!

CHAPTER SIX: ENVIRONMENTAL FACTORS

There are certain things you can control your exposure to and those you cannot control. You need to be aware of these exposures and avoid them as much as possible before you conceive, during pregnancy, and after. Often there are natural options available that work well and will be safer for you and your family. Take a look at what you use and come in contact with, and be sure it is natural and nontoxic as often as possible. Please do not take the information I am about to share as advice to hibernate! I just want you to be aware, so you can consciously limit exposure to environmental toxins.

Pesticides

One environmental toxin to avoid is pesticide. There are many dangers associated with the chemicals used for a weed-free, green lawn. Like many other toxins, these pose a health threat to developing eggs and baby. Breathing in fumes can be harmful, and many fumes can linger for days or even weeks, depending on how strong the pesticides are. Be aware if you live near a golf course or have neighbors who are using harmful chemical pesticides and fertilizers in their lawns, too. Most people like to open the windows when spring approaches, but depending on which chemicals are used in your neighborhood, this may not be the best idea. If you smell something like a chemical or ammonia smell, you can be sure it is toxic. You may also see signs posted in lawns saying not to go in the lawn for a certain time after pesticides are applied. Look for signs that have a skull and crossbones pictured (since this indicates danger).

If I was trying to conceive or already pregnant, I would not sit in grass that has been treated with these kinds of chemicals even months after application. Needless to say my children do not play in such grass. When trying to conceive, avoid lawns or park areas that may be toxic. You will have to check with your local municipality as to if they use toxic products in parks or public spaces. As more is becoming known about pesticide toxicity, many golf courses have switched to greener, nontoxic methods. Look into what they use in your area—it pays to be safe.

Fragrance

The next environmental culprit to avoid is fragrance from laundry detergents, air fresheners, baby products—you name it! This is hard to avoid in some cases. Avoiding fragrances entirely can be difficult. Often we must share cramped, common "air space" on airplanes, subways or trains, movie theaters, or in churches. Some days it seems impossible to avoid those men or women who find the need to take a bath in their favorite perfume or cologne. What they do not know is how bad the synthetic chemicals in the products are for them and those forced to breathe in their fragrance.

Laundry detergent and fabric softener also can contain harmful fragrances. If you live near a Laundromat, moving is an option. If you must use a Laundromat, consider having someone else do the laundry. (I even wonder about the build-up in the public machines from others using the Laundromat. It seems easy for the fragrance from other people's laundry products to end up affecting the smell of your clothes.) If you have the space and finances, invest in your own washer and dryer.

Another culprit is the air freshener used in the majority of public bathrooms. Many of the chemicals found in synthetic fragrances, including phthalates, are endocrine disruptors. Even a slight hormonal imbalance can throw off your ability to conceive. Sometimes it is hard to avoid when you "Gotta go… Gotta go... RIGHT NOW!" in the last trimester of pregnancy. All you can do is hold your breath and be very quick about your business!

I find the fragrance used in many baby diapers to be annoying! Babies poop, it is a fact of parenthood. Why do companies try to cover it up by putting fragrance in the diapers? They are exposing our babies to toxins, which I believe should be outlawed! My favorite diaper thus far is from the Honest Company, which has no fragrance, is nontoxic and biodegradable. Nature Babycare (Naty) is also free of toxins and biodegradable and I used their diapers with my first baby. Another option is cloth diapers from a diaper service. Just investigate which chemicals they use to clean them. Of course, you can clean the cloth diapers yourself, if you have time and patience. It is a money saver, but not for everyone. As far as swim diapers go, Iplay makes awesome reusable swim diapers, which we have used for years because they wash up very easily. No fragrant diapers allowed please!

Fragrances are hidden in various baby products all the time, too. Walk down the aisles of a baby store and see for yourself how many toxins are lingering in the air. From plastic baby seats to plastic toys, companies seem to think that adding fragrance to their products will make them more appealing. For some reason, they think it's better to cover up the smell of your baby's spit up or other mess. Clearly, they have not seen the research on endocrine disruptors or they would not put them in their products.

What you can do, when registering for baby gifts or purchasing items for friends or family, is have your husband do "the sniff test." If it has a fragrance, even a mild one, do not put it on your registry or buy it. You do not want anyone's baby to inhale chemical, synthetic smells—no matter how great the product. When opting for an all-natural, green lifestyle, choose items made from wood, wool, and cotton. There is even a bamboo potty seat on the market! These toys and baby items are typically free of scents or use natural, essential oils to add fragrance.

Paint Fumes

Paint fumes contain volatile organic compounds (VOC)—an important environmental toxin to avoid. Today, there are healthier paints to choose from, such as no-VOC or Green Guard Certified paints like Mythic paint and Sherwin- Williams. Most people want to paint the nursery before the baby comes, but if you can wait, it is best. If you must redecorate, use a safe paint and have someone else do the job. Open plenty of windows for good ventilation, while painting. Better yet, go out of town or stay with family and friends for a few days, while the job is being done. A pregnant mom (or a woman trying to get pregnant) should not be exposed to the dust and mess from construction or the unknown compounds that are emitted into the air when updating your home. No one should really be exposed to these toxins either.

If you are planning to move, think twice if you are considering moving to an apartment building. Most buildings use standard paints, which are toxic. In some cases moving is unavoidable, just be aware and open windows to air out any toxins in your new space. Having plants in your home like the spider plant or aloe plant can help clean the toxins in the air.

Automobile and Transportation Toxins

Although everyone has to service their car from time to time, it is not necessary to wait in the garage and be exposed to any of the many carcinogens that could be lurking there. Gas fumes are toxic, and most windshield washer fluid comes with a warning label, for example. Brake dust from the streets fills the air near busy streets or highways. Use caution when dining at a sidewalk café and be sure to have silverware clean of any dust from the street. Exhaust fumes from cars, buses, trucks and diesel trains can make their way into the air you breathe. As you travel down the highway behind a smelly truck, keep the windows up. Newly tarred or blacktopped parking lots and roads should be avoided, too. Keep away from places and things that have these smells, the toxins emitted from them that go into the air are extremely harmful. When buying a car, a used one is much safer as it has off-gased some of the toxins. That new car smell means it is toxic. The many toxins associated with transportation are great. Some of these you may never have thought about. When you add them all up, the exposure is much more than you would have realized. It becomes more evident that being green as far as transportation goes, is a must!

Electronic Devices and EMFs

Radiation from cell phones and laptops are another common cause of low sperm count. Keep the phone out of your pocket, and the laptop on the desk. Radiation from your phone can cause problems with your thyroid, which in turn affects all the systems of the body. Even though the levels of radiation are low, the heat and radiation emitted affect sperm count in the same way that wearing-tight fitting briefs heat up the pants and sperm. Although I know of no conclusive research, I am concerned that radiation from electronic devices can also affect egg health. Wi-fi for computers is another issue and even banned in some schools in Europe. Think of all the waves going into the air, no one really knows what they are doing or how they are truly affecting us.

What these devices have in come is their Electromagnetic frequencies or EMFs. This is something we should become more aware of since our daily exposure is more than we may realize. These include overhead power lines and cell towers. We cannot forget the radiation from our television, refrigerators, computers, printers, and other various appliances throughout our homes or workplaces that emit EMFs. While we can choose to live in an area with fewer overhead power lines, the items in our homes have become a necessity.

There are steps you can take to reduce your exposure and support your health. You can start by diffusing or applying Young Living rosemary oil to your feet or drink rosemary tea. Natural stones like Hematite and Black Tourmaline are protective. There are also items on the market which can reduce exposure like bracelets, necklaces and pendants. There are many options out there. You should get electronics out the bedroom for sure. There is also a paint you can apply to the walls which can limit exposure from room to room. Protecting yourself from EMFs may seem impossible but you will be healthier after doing so.

Smoke and BBQs

While I think it is a no-brainer, people still do not realize that there is secondhand smoke, and now third hand smoke which accumulates on surfaces where someone smokes. Smoke should be avoided, and not just by those trying to conceive. This includes smoke from campfires and even your cozy, winter fire in the fireplace. While they may seem inviting, the toxins emitted could pose a risk, depending on what is burning. Wood smoke and cigarette smoke are similar—both are carcinogenic. Before you light a fire to create a little romance, think again. The smoke from fireworks displays are a concern, too. Leave any areas where you may be exposed, like downwind of a fireworks display!

Smoke from that summer BBQ can be just as much of a hazard— not to mention the charbroiled burgers with black around the edges. Those grill marks on meat and char-grilled hot dogs may be tasty, but they also may be bad for your health. Whenever the meats are cooked for long periods of time at high temperatures, they can form certain chemicals that are carcinogenic. There are some things you can do while grilling to lower the exposure of toxins. You can marinate your food, which seems to protect the meat. Opt for chicken or veggies on the grill rather than fattier meats such as beef or pork.

Another chemical reaction happens as meat juices drop to the bottom of the grill, creating even more toxic gases to circulate around your dinner steak. If you must have that steak on the grill every once in a blue moon, flip it instead of pricking it with a fork. Use a thermometer so you don't overcook or leave the food on the grill any longer than necessary.

Most importantly, keep your grill clean! Those charred crumbs of mystery meat left on the grill will reheat and release more chemicals. Start with a clean grill before each BBQ to ensure you are not increasing toxin exposure. This from AOL Health: "A 2003 study conducted by a French environmental campaigning group Robin des Bois found that the average two-hour barbecue can release about the same level of dioxins, a group of chemicals linked to the increased risk of cancer, as 220,000 cigarettes. Cooking on an elevated rack to allow fat to drip away helps further reduce exposure to dioxins, suggests the Illinois Department of Public Health."

Have I totally ruined your idea of a summer BBQ? Just be cautious. Don't eat blackened or charred foods. It is especially important for your young children or for those men and women trying to conceive a child not to have them. You do not want anything toxic going in your body during this delicate time. Women breastfeeding should use caution as well when ingesting food from a BBQ. The studies speak for themselves.

Pets

Pets can be a joyous addition to the family. Pets are our "first babies," and we love to cuddle with them and put our faces in their fur. But think about what you are putting on them, because it gets into the air you breathe. If you are bathing them with a common pet shampoo, you are exposing yourself and them to unhealthy chemicals. The pet groomers also have fragrant shampoos and sprays to make "Fluffie" or "Fido" fresh and clean. They are most likely just as toxic, and the scents can be nauseating.

If treating your pets with toxic flea and tick repellant, you are exposing them and yourself to hidden dangers. We all want to keep fleas and ticks from coming into our homes, especially if we live in an area where the ticks carry Lyme's disease. Go for natural alternatives, which are more readily available these days. Essential oil combinations like Purification or just Citronella oil are great to help pets enjoy the outdoors annoyance free and smell fresh. You can find these from Young Living or make your own outdoor collar for your pet.

Outdoor Collar Recipe

Young Living Oils:

1 drop Cedarwood
3 drops Purification
2 drops Lavender

2 drops Citronella
3 drops Citrus Fresh

Mix in a stainless steel bowl, soak natural fiber collar in oil and let dry. There are many recipes you can find online.

If you are trying to keep pests out of your home there are natural alternatives that also use essential oils, and various recipes you can find online to repel just about any pest. From mosquitoes and ants to spiders and flies, there is a recipe to repel them that does not use toxic ingredients.

Lead

You may think lead is only in paint. It can be found in other sources, as I already mentioned, such as china. You can also find it in holiday decorations, such as Christmas lights, your artificial Christmas tree, garland, or the paint on your ceramic Nativity scene. It can also be in other holiday decorations and ornaments. Most cheaply made items usually contain some sort of hazard and are usually imported, so you have no idea what they have come in contact with on their way to your home. Lead can also be found in kid's plastic jewelry and also in the ink of books printed before 1985. Be aware when you are handling such items, and wash your hands afterwards or wear gloves!

Wrinkle Free Clothes

Wrinkle free clothes and sheets are another hidden danger. When you are trying to conceive, you may be unknowingly breathing in toxins from your wrinkle free clothes or while rolling around on wrinkle free sheets trying to make that baby. I joke, but seriously this is a hazard no one warns you about. What is worse, you bring that new baby home and the last thing you want to do is iron your husband's clothes while the baby naps right? So you think, why not buy some wrinkle-free shirts and pants, and maybe a few sheets? Wrong! This is the last thing you ever want to bring into your home. These items contain formaldehyde to give them that crisp look. It is a human carcinogen. Need I say more? Think about how this chemical could affect your sperm and eggs!

A few years back, 180 items were tested. A *New York Times* article reported: "About 5.5 percent of the items—primarily wrinkle-free shirts and pants, easy-care pillow cases, crib sheets, and a boy's baseball hat—exceeded the most stringent standards of 75 parts per million, for products that touch the skin. (Levels must be undetectable, or less than 20 parts per million for children under three years, and can be as high as 300 parts per million for products like outerwear that do not come into direct contact with the skin.)"

Just think what happens when your husband is burping the baby in his wrinkle-free shirt or what baby is breathing as you place him/her on toxic sheets. You may not know it but formaldehyde is hiding is many household items, like your upholstered sofa, curtains, and the construction materials in your walls. Although you cannot avoid everything, you can limit your exposure by choosing not to buy wrinkle-free, wrinkle-resistant, no iron, or permanent press items. Organic cotton, bamboo, and wool are your safest option for clothes and sheets, plus they are becoming more readily available. If you cannot find them, look for ones that are not "Wrinkle Free" or "Easy Care".

BPA, Plastics, and Food Packaging

Most of us have heard that BPA is found in bottles and plastic food packaging. But have you heard that there is BPA in your cash register receipt? Receipts. Receipts. Receipts. As you go through your varied receipts at tax time in hopes of getting a big refund, wear gloves or wash your hands constantly. BPA, which is short for Bisphenol A, is an industrial chemical used to make plastic. After you touch the receipts you do not want this BPA ink transferring to your children, your mouth, your food, or anywhere else. BPA is now banned in baby bottles. Until BPA is banned everywhere, handle receipts with caution, especially if you are trying to conceive.

Another toxin most people don't think about is food packaging. Avoid canned foods with BPA lining as well. One chemical called perfluorooctanoic acid (PFOA) is in the lining of microwave popcorn bags, candy wrappers, fast food wrappers, and pizza boxes. It is a synthetic chemical that can increase the risk of infertility. Another reason we should not eat fast food.

Chlorine and Chlorinated Pools

While we are told that small amounts of chlorine may be OK, no one knows how much is too much. Chlorine is widely used to kill bacteria in drinking water and in swimming pools, and is also found in cleaning products. While there is no concrete research that shows swimming in chlorine can be harmful to a baby, we do know that chlorine can be toxic if exposed to in high amounts. Consider the amount of chlorine your body is exposed to, especially if you are an avid swimmer or your water supply is highly chlorinated. The fetus is highly sensitive to chemical exposures, and chlorine is a chemical.

We can usually recognize the smell of a highly-chlorinated pool. This is very apparent with indoor pools and highly-trafficked public pools. Exposure to chlorine can come from chlorine gas or from contact with water. If swimming is something you love, an outdoor pool that is properly chlorinated is probably your best choice as well as waiting to swim until the third trimester. This way you won't inhale any fumes that are trapped in a building.

Scientists in the UK suggest that chlorine exposure via mother to unborn baby could increase risk of allergies and asthma, and therefore change their immune systems. Scientists from St. Johns Institute of Dermatology in London and the University of Manchester are doing further research on chemical exposure during the critical window of pregnancy.

Before you conceive, reconsider your environmental exposures to chlorine. If you are a swimmer, maybe it is a good idea to take a break or limit swimming, so you don't expose yourself to high amounts of chlorine. Until further research is done on chlorine and possible links to birth defects, allergies, asthma, or even miscarriage, swim with caution and filter your water. After you swim, bathe with soap and water rather than just rinsing off the chlorinated water. Try to avoid swimming on days when the pool has been serviced, because it most likely has fresh chemicals.

British researchers have also found that a chemical by-product of chlorine called trihalomethane (THMs), which is found in very high levels in swimming pools, may also be hazardous for pregnant women and their unborn babies. Study author Mark J. Nieuwenhuijsen, PhD, an environmental science researcher at Imperial College of Science, Technology, and Medicine in London, noted that levels of THMs were considerably higher in swimming pools than in tap water.

"Miscarriage, low birth weight, neural tube defects, urinary tract defects, and other [medical issues] have been associated with exposure to THMs, but the evidence so far has been inconsistent and inconclusive," writes Nieuwenhuijsen.

After reading this, do you think it is safe to swim during pre-pregnancy while trying to conceive or in the first or second trimester? You can decide for yourself. Another study concluded: "In tests, pools were found to have 'relatively high' levels of the disinfectant by-products, which have been linked to reproductive problems. A one-hour swim was found to give a chloroform dose 141 times higher than a ten-minute shower."

This is a scary thought for a developing egg, sperm or fetus. Clearly more conclusive research is needed or everyone should be swimming in saltwater or ionized pools, or at clean beaches. Decide what is right for you. Swimming is a great exercise—just use caution. Avoid highly populated pools, indoor pools, and pools that are not well ventilated. Also, shower before you swim to remove organic matter that will react with chlorine. Shower after a swim with soap.

The signs of chlorine exposure are burning eyes, nose, and throat, which most of us have experienced after swimming in a pool with too much chlorine. Coughing, tightness in the chest, difficulty breathing, and shortness of breath are all common signs of high chlorine exposure.

Watery eyes, wheezing, nausea, vomiting, and blurred vision can also occur.

If you have a chlorinated pool and want a safer option, you can convert your pool to salt water. An even better option is ionization, which uses copper, zinc and silver to treat the water. Hiring a company who specializes in this type of conversion for your pool will be well worth it. You will want your future children swimming in healthy chemical-free water! It is the greenest option as well!

Fluoride

Whether the Fluoride is safe, is a big debate among people. Some people are convinced we need it to prevent cavities, while others are dead set against it being added to water supplies or given in supplements to kids. Fluoride is added to some public drinking water supplies and in numerous brands of toothpastes. It is also found in some drugs, like anesthetics, antacids, anti-anxiety, antibiotics, antidepressants, anti-fungal antibiotics, and antihistamines. If you are on any of these you should work with a doctor to eliminate them at least three months prior to trying to conceive. The amount of Fluoride we are exposed to in everyday life is high naturally, so removing unnecessary supplements or medications containing fluoride should be considered, especially if there are natural alternatives. Fluoride makes its way into our food supply through watering of crops and processing of foods, too. Plus, drinking large amounts of tea can increase fluoride levels in the body, as can consuming wine or grape juice made in the US.

Fluoride is a neurotoxin, which has been linked to many diseases. It has been added to drinking water since the 50's. Fluoride also suppresses thyroid function and can destroy enzymes. In 1955, the *New England Journal of Medicine* reported a 400% increase in the number of thyroid cancer cases in the years after San Francisco's water began to be fluoridated.

Fluoride can have an effect on fetal brain development, too, if fluoride poisoning occurs. In fact, studies done in China "found evidence of significant neurological damage, including neuronal degeneration and reduced levels of neurotransmitters such as norepinephrine" In the 1960s the FDA banned the use of prenatal fluoride due to concern that it could affect the unborn baby. We know that infants should not be exposed to fluoride, because they do not have the ability to excrete it from their kidneys. Studies also indicate fluoride can lower IQ, because it can affect the blood brain barrier, and lead to low birth weight and premature birth.

One study published in *Current Science* noted that pregnant women with high levels of fluoride suffered greater risk for iron deficient anemia (Susheela, 2010). This study also noted that fluoride decreases nutrients that are especially needed for a healthy pregnancy and birth by reducing the amount of red blood cells, blocking good gut bacteria, and inhibiting vitamin B-12 production in the mother's body. Learn more at: www.healingourchildren.org/the-fluoride-deception-pregnancy-and-childhood

Fluoride is still added to some drinking water and encouraged by some dentists. Safe levels have not been determined and, since everyone's tolerance is different, it may be best to eliminate fluoride as much as possible. There is much more information to be found at www.fluoridealert.org. The studies speak for themselves, but even if they were inconclusive wouldn't you rather be safe than sorry?

Mercury

Mercury is a naturally occurring element found in nature. Mercury is dangerous for anyone in elevated amounts, but especially for those trying to conceive. It can affect the nervous system of unborn babies, and affect the heart, brain, lungs, kidneys, and immune system. It can be found in thermometers, light switches, and coal. When coal is burned, it releases the largest amount of mercury into the air, which then settles on nearby land and water—not the best thing for the environment or the animals feeding nearby. Mercury can also be found in button cell batteries, dental amalgam fillings, fluorescent light bulbs, and the vaccine preservative Thimerosal.

Hopefully, most people have read or seen the warnings on consuming fish that are high in mercury. To recap, the fish that should be avoided are Ahi Tuna, Shark, King Mackerel, Marlin, Orange Roughy, Tilefish, Swordfish, Chilean Sea Bass, Bluefish, Grouper, Spanish or Gulf Mackerel, Albacore canned Tuna, and Yellowfin Tuna to start. Refer back to the chapter on Diet for the complete list.

Compact fluorescent lights (CFLs) may be good for saving energy, but when they break mercury vapors escape into the air. When it comes to CFLs, don't buy them anymore. This also goes for mercury thermometers, too. Digital thermometers are easy to use and pretty accurate. Though button cell batteries do not require recycling, be aware that they do contain mercury should its outer layer becomes compromised.

Before you choose to vaccinate, do your research and ask other Moms pro-vax and anti-vax how their children reacted to mercury and chemicals in vaccines and their other ingredients. Watch the movie, *The Greater Good* and truly inform yourself of all the risks. Look into what each vaccine is truly for and if it will benefit your child. Many religions are against vaccinating for various reasons. Only you can decide how to care for you and your baby's body that God has created. Think long and hard on your choices. Pray for the wisdom to protect your health in a way you feel is best. If your child has an MTHFR gene mutation, the toxins will not be the best choice. This is a very personal decision and lots of heated arguments ensue all the time on this topic. Do what you feel is best for your family and be informed. Ask the doctor for the vaccines that do not contain Thimerosal if you do choose vaccinations. These vaccines are available, and though you may trouble the doctor to obtain them, it is your choice. Be aware the flu vaccine does contain Thimerosal, too. Also, I would NEVER get a vaccine myself when pregnant no matter what the doctor says. There have been no proper tests for safety.

Next we move on to dental amalgam fillings as a cause of concern for our health. There is an older group of people who have had mercury fillings for years without health issues. There is also an array of people who have mercury fillings and have suffered from poor health due to mercury exposure. I wonder why this is the case. Are some people better at eliminating toxins? Has the quality and amount of mercury in the fillings changed over the decades?

Since there are safer options for filling cavities, opt for those. If you do have mercury fillings, you can have them removed by a qualified holistic dentist. Some people feel that if they are in good condition, you can leave them alone until they need to be removed. This is a personal choice, depending on the health of your teeth and condition of your fillings. Replacing your mercury fillings can be a costly undertaking, depending on how many you have in your mouth. You may also look for a mercury-free dentist so you are not exposed to mercury in the office. Not all dentists know how to properly handle teeth with mercury. There is a safe way for removal and working on them so no one gets exposed. Mercury vapors can get released just by chewing or brushing your teeth! Check out holisticdental.org or hg-free.com for more information.

Be aware that if you are trying to conceive, you may want to wait to have them removed if there are any signs of filling deterioration. While the qualified dentists can limit your exposure during removal of mercury, there still may be a minimal amount of mercury you are exposed to. If you are pregnant, do not get them removed until after you are done breastfeeding.

We conceived our first child about eight months after my husband had the majority of his mercury fillings removed. I have no mercury fillings as I was blessed with healthy teeth and had my first cavity at 26. Whatever the condition of your teeth and fillings are, be sure to see a dentist well before trying to conceive in order to limit mercury exposure.

The list of environmental toxins to avoid are long, but you will breathe a lot easier when you start to limit your exposures. You may now feel like you should move to a deserted island to avoid them. That may not be a viable option for all, so just avoid them! Some people get headaches, nausea or other symptoms like rashes and are not sure why. Environmental toxins could be the reason. Being aware of your environment can help you detect what is truly ailing you.

CHAPTER SEVEN: FENG SHUI FOR FERTILITY AND DE-CLUTTERING YOUR HOME

In Chinese medicine, when energy—also known as chi—is blocked or stagnant in the body, it can result in poor health. In Asian cultures, blockages in the physical environments, where we live and work, can also create imbalances in our health or in other areas of our lives. *Feng shui* is an ancient Chinese practice, which involves placing items in your home in a way that maximizes the flow of energy. In turn, this fresh infusion can bring prosperity, health, peace of mind, safety, love, good relationships, and even new family members into your life.

Before you conceive, you will want to consider your home environment for various reasons, including how the flow of energy is affected by your current surroundings. We want positive free-flowing energy in our lives that ensures a balance of yin and yang. Yin and yang are one of the most basic concepts in Chinese Medicine—positives and negatives that coexist side-by-side in nature. Yin is female and passive, while yang is male and aggressive. Although they are opposites, one cannot exist without the other. By creating balance of yin and yang, you will allow room for a new life. Your home should be a place of peace and sanctuary, where you come to relax, rest, and regroup. This will be the perfect environment for a new baby.

Decluttering

When your home is cluttered, it can make you feel stressed and uneasy. These kinds of emotions can create unpleasant physiological changes in the body—picture the opposite of "feel-good hormones" flowing through your system. Searching for the things you need wastes time, energy, and often money. How many times have you purchased another item, simply because you couldn't find the one you already had? Further, having items you do not need can make your home feel crowded. Most importantly, they take up space, which limits the new people, things, and experiences you can bring into your life.

Removing clutter before you conceive is a good way to create positive energy in your home. Are you a hoarder or a closet packrat? Is your home organized, with every item in its proper place? Or do you spend half an hour searching for your favorite pair of jeans in the piles of clothes that are scattered all over your bedroom? When it's time to leave for work, to do an art project with your child, or to take the family on a fun outing, does it take forever to find everything you need or to get out the door?

Items should be easy to find. Being a parent can be chaotic at the best of times, so knowing where things are and putting things in a designated place are two simple ways to create a support structure for yourself and your family.

Getting organized and getting rid of things is another way of going green. Many items can be reused, recycled, or upcycled. Consider those clothes you have not worn in a few years, the books you planned to read but never make time for, and the gifts from your Aunt (which really aren't your taste). Donate old items to a charity, school, or library. Let friends shop your closet! Your trash can easily become someone else's treasure.

Practicing Feng Shui for Fertility

There are many schools of Feng Shui, but all focus on where you place certain items within your home. Some schools also consider the direction—north, south, east, west—that a room or items in that room, such as a bed, face. If you would like to prepare yourself and your home for conception using some basic Feng Shui principles, here are some suggestions:

Clutter

- Make sure the area around your front door is free of clutter, clean, and inviting. Energy can easily flow into your home this way. Also, take note if anything outside is blocking your front door, such as a tree, car, or a garbage can. Moving these items will increase the flow of energy into your home.
- From time to time, visit the places in your house that tend to collect clutter, knowing that you will need to reorganize and to make sure that children's hands don't have access to certain things.

Placement

- If you want to create positive or creative fertility energy, take a look at the west side of your home. The west side is associated with children, so take a look at the rooms on the west side of your home. Similarly, the west side of each individual room in your house is associated with children. You want these areas to be free from clutter and organized.
- The male should sleep with his head pointing northwest. He should also work and eat facing northwest. The woman should sleep on the right side of the bed with the man on the left.
- If there is a bathroom on the west side of the home, be sure to keep the door closed.

Location

- Make sure your bed does not share a wall with a door, bathroom, or kitchen.
- If you have a ceiling fan above your bed then it is time to go shopping for a new light for the bedroom. In Feng Shui, it is believed that having a fan slice through the air above you also cuts through the energy of the abdomen.

- Televisions, computers, exercise equipment, books, mirrors, and plants should also be removed if they are in your bedroom. These items take away good Feng Shui energy. The bedroom should have yin energy (female), not the yang (male) of all the mentioned items. If you must have a few of these items, keep them in a cabinet so they are hidden.

Symbols

There are also symbols used in Feng Shui such as dragons, elephants, double fish, red paper lanterns, and a single piece of hollow bamboo, which are all thought to boost fertility.

- Make a red paper lantern and hang it by the bed.
- Place a small dragon on your husband's side of the bed.
- Place one of these figurines on the west side of the home to promote fertility. If you chose an elephant figurine or photo, be sure the trunk is down so the energy is stored and accumulates.
- Place pictures of baby animals or babies around the home.
- Place pomegranates, another fertility symbol, in your home. You can buy them to eat, place them in a bowl for decoration, or have pictures of pomegranates in your kitchen or elsewhere in your home.

Feng Shui for Existing and Future Children's Rooms

- Having kids jump on your bed is also said to create baby energy! If you don't have any yet…borrow some from family and friends, and have them jump away!
- If you are planning to put your child in a room that is already occupied, you will want to remove any items you have no need for. Again, this allows you to make room for a new life and for the new essential items your baby will need.
- Just because I suggest you de-clutter, do not turn around and restock your home with every baby gadget on the market! That

is actually the opposite of what your baby (or toddler) needs. Plus, limiting the number of items in the nursery will help you keep his belongings tidy until he can learn to put his toys away himself.

Simplicity Parenting by Kim John Payne is a great book to read during your pregnancy. In fact, I think it is a must for parents and grandparents because it discusses the pitfalls of overbuying, over-stimulating, and overstocking. Living in excess with your new baby is not good for either of you.

When my husband and I wanted to conceive our third child, I noticed that the west side of our home was very cluttered with things that we were storing in a back hallway. Going through what was there and de-cluttering not only opened the fertility gates for us, it also gave us a feeling of peace as a result of being more organized. We also made a red paper lantern to hang beside the bed and placed pictures of our other two children around the home. Our third baby was the easiest to conceive! If you believe in Chinese medicine like acupuncture, then these tips may help you, too. Try a few for fun and remove the things that may hinder your chances of conception. Even if you are a bit skeptical, what have you got to lose? Living in a de-cluttered and organized home will make you feel good, like it did us, and that is a great first step toward conceiving.

CHAPTER EIGHT: ALKALINE VS. ACIDIC DIET AND PLANNING FOR A BOY OR GIRL

Could diet influence your chance of conceiving a boy or a girl? We know having a healthy diet is critical to a healthy pregnancy. If you have the time and dedication to take it one step further—you can try to influence the sex of the baby by following a strict alkaline or acid diet. Although the medical community has not produced a lot of research on this topic, there are those that swear it works. One of the few studies supporting the claim that diet can affect a baby's gender was a study done in the Netherlands from 2001-2006. In this study, couples used an acidic diet and timing to try to conceive a girl, after having boys. The results are very clear from CBS Statistics Netherlands on the Dutch population: Women who followed the diet and did the timing correctly had a greater likelihood of having a girl. This study is a great indicator that sex selection can be achieved naturally, if mothers follow proper diet and timing.

In 2008, a team of researchers headed by Dr. Fiona Mathews of Exeter University conducted a study on whether alkaline diets affect the chances of conceiving a boy. Turns out, what was once considered an old wives tale, may now have scientific validity. The studies show that eating an alkaline diet makes the cervical fluid less acidic, which creates a better environment for the survival of male sperm.

Also, while some foods are naturally acidic, when they are consumed and in the blood, they become alkaline. Lemons, for instance, shift from acidic to alkaline when consumed and absorbed into the bloodstream.

You can get a pH testing kit to see if you are currently more acidic or alkaline before you change your diet.

Alkaline Diet for Boys

If attempting an alkaline diet with hopes for a baby boy, avoid dairy, sugar, breads, pastas, wheat products, legumes, corn and corn products, blueberries, and processed foods. These foods are highly acidic. You can add dairy, bread, pasta, legumes, corn, and blueberries back to your diet *after* you conceive. Take note that if you do follow a gluten-free diet, many of the substitute flours can be acidic. Check ingredients carefully, or make your own bread. A diet rich in potassium and sodium (but not too high) will also make the body more alkaline. If you have high blood pressure, consult your doctor, as increasing sodium intake is not recommended. Sea salt or pink himalayan are the best form of salts. Drinking lemon water will also help make the body alkaline. It is crucial to never skip breakfast and to increase your calorie intake by about 400 calories if you are currently on a normal caloric intake. Skipping breakfast can decrease your blood glucose levels as well. Eating the following foods organic and non-GMO is your best option when available.

Alkaline foods you want to consume:

Fruits: ripe bananas, cherries, pineapple, watermelon, apples, pears, kiwi, grapes, berries, avocados

Vegetables: Brussels sprouts, celery, asparagus, artichoke, broccoli, spinach, cucumber, cauliflower, carrots, all leafy greens preferably blanched or cooked, baked potatoes, sweet potatoes, pumpkin, onions, garlic, ginger, leeks, cabbages, bok choy, kale, cilantro, zucchini, green beans

Nuts: almonds, pumpkin seeds

Pickles: (high sodium content)

Red meat: once a week

Use apple cider vinegar instead of red wine vinegars or white vinegar. In addition, the fruits must be at room temperature or cooked (think baked apples). In Chinese medicine, cooked foods are better for conception. Eating a lot of raw foods is not advised. A lot of these foods can be made into soups or put in a bone broth, which is also healing. Increasing your overall intake of vegetables, except corn, easily makes your diet more alkaline. I also do not recommend dried fruits, since they can increase blood sugar levels too much. Brushing your teeth with baking soda is also an option if you want to change your pH balance.

Since you should not be skipping breakfast, and most cereals are acidic, you have options. You can have egg whites instead of the whole egg. Or, balance the meal out and have a spinach omelet instead. The yolk of the egg is acidic. You can also try this Kale Smoothie Recipe.

Kale Smoothie Recipe

Serves 2

This is a great smoothie for breakfast or a snack. You can save excess in the refrigerator for one day. It may dry up a little but you can add almond milk to the smoothie to make it fresh again.

Ingredients:

3-4 leaves of Organic Kale Blanched
4 Tablespoons Organic Hemp Powder
3 Tablespoons Organic Chia Powder
1 teaspoon Maca Powder (Fertility boosting)
1 teaspoon or less of Green Powder Stevia (depends on how sweet you prefer)
1 Banana
2 Tablespoons or more of Organic Raw Almond Butter
2 Tablespoons Organic Raw Cacao Powder (a superfood)
Organic Almond Milk (365 Brand does not contain Carrageenan)

1 teaspoon Flax Oil or 1 Tablespoon ground Flax Seeds (reduces inflammation/grind seeds in coffee grinder, fresher is best)
Add ½ -1 teaspoon Chlorella Powder (optional)

Directions:

1. Wash the kale and remove the leafy part, throw out the hard stem, put the leaves in the high-powered blender. If the blender is glass, add hot water to cover. If it is plastic, blanche the leaves in hot water just so they brighten in color a bit.
2. Blend well.
3. Add other ingredients, except almond milk.
4. Add almond milk a little at a time to get desired smoothie consistency.
5. Add ice if needed.

Note: Warm smoothies are good for conception. If they come out too hot, you only need to add a few ice cubes to get them a little chilled or to room temp. The idea is warm, never cold or frozen. If you are trying for a girl, you can omit the kale or add Goat Yogurt to the mix for variation. Substitute berries instead of banana.

Acidic Diet for Girls

If you are trying for a girl, you want to eat an acidic diet. Include lots of organic dairy products like low sodium cheeses, yogurt, and milk. Calcium-rich foods are ideal along with magnesium, so load up on broccoli and leafy greens. You can have pasta and breads in moderation. Eat more grains like quinoa, rice (in moderation if it is jasmine or low risk for arsenic), and buckwheat. Gluten-free may be better if you are battling fertility issues such as PCOS. Since corn is acidic you can have organic/GMO-free corn products. So indulge in some homemade Mexican enchiladas, nachos, or tacos. You can eat all types of beans and lentils as well. Eat eggs with the yolks, which are acidic. You will love that you can have chocolate on the acidic diet! Organic dark is best with over 70% cacao.

Fruits: prunes, plums, cranberries, grapefruit, tamarind, blueberries, strawberries

Vegetables: squash, corn, lentils, olives, broccoli, swiss chard, spinach, kale, dandelion greens

Nuts: cashew, peanuts, walnuts, pecans, legumes

Meat: beef, liver, shellfish, tuna, sardines

Dairy: butter, cheese, yogurt

Oil: avocado oil, sunflower oil, olive oil, sesame oil

Grains: buckwheat, oats, brown rice, quinoa

Avoid foods high in potassium like bananas, potatoes, and lower your sodium intake. Also, avoid apples, almonds, and mushrooms.

Timing Affects the Sex Too

If you know you want to try for a certain sex and have chosen the proper diet, it is time to take a closer look at the timing of sex. "The Shettles Method" can help you determine exactly when you should have sex based on the preferred gender. First, lets get the facts straight: The female sperm are very strong, live longer than male sperm, and swim slow. The male sperm are very quick, but they die off quickly. How does this affect your chances of conceiving a boy or a girl? Arming yourself with all the information, will help you know what to do and when!

If you are trying for a boy, for example, refrain from having sex (or use a condom when having sex!) the closer you get to ovulation. If your partner does not deposit sperm in the vagina prior to ovulation and waits until the day of or the day before ovulation, your chance of conceiving a boy is much greater. Because male sperm die quickly, if you have sex too soon before ovulation, there is a greater chance that the male sperm will die off before your egg is released. Since the majority of female sperm survive longer, most likely, they will win the race if you have sex before ovulation.

On the other hand, if you are trying for a girl, you can have unprotected sex for days leading up to your ovulation day. It is good to stop at about two to three days before you think you will ovulate.

Trying for a girl is a little harder. Especially if you have an irregular cycle, because pinpointing when to stop having sex can be an issue. So, chart your menstrual cycle for a few months to get an idea of which day of your cycle you ovulate. When you have a lot of egg white cervical mucus, you are either ovulating or just finished ovulating. Having unprotected sex at this time, you are more likely to conceive a boy. Whereas, if you have sex a few days before ovulation, the female sperm have an advantage.

Diet and timing together will give you the greatest chance of getting the results you want.

Pinpointing Ovulation

By the way, you may not ovulate on the same day every month. Some women believe it is on day 14, but the truth is, that is an average number. Some women can ovulate very early in the cycle or very late. Please note, ovulating too early or too late can also indicate hormonal issues. Always consult your doctor if you think you might have a medical problem. If you ovulate too early, for example, the egg may not be mature enough for conception. If ovulation is too late, on the other hand, the egg may be "old" to sustain itself long enough to implant. Not to worry, though: Women have had successful pregnancies ovulating very early and very late. Simple awareness of your body and when you typically ovulate is important, because outside factors like stress or illness can throw off your ovulation for a month.

So how do you know when you are ovulating or not? You must chart your cycle. To start, you will need a basal body thermometer, which you can purchase at a pharmacy. This special thermometer allows you to detect your body temperature when you rise in the morning. You should take your temperature before you get out of bed each morning. Leaving the thermometer under your pillow or in your nightstand is best so you do not move much before rising—this will give you the most accurate reading.

Temperature readings can also be affected by too little sleep, illness, alcohol consumption, and outside temperatures as winter comes. Do not drink anything before you test. The best day to start testing is the first day of your period. Your temperature will most likely be 97.5-97.9 when you have your period and stay in a similar range up until you ovulate. The numbers will naturally go up and down a little each day. Typically, just one day prior to ovulation, your temperature will suddenly drop. Then, the next day it will spike up past 98.0. Some women do not experience the drop then spike, just the spike. This spike in temperature indicates that you have ovulated. Your temperature should remain high for the rest of your cycle until you get your next period or you get a positive result on a pregnancy test. If your temperature fluctuates too much—meaning it drops below 98 at the time of ovulation or later in your cycle—your hormones may be off that month and you will not conceive. Chart again the following month or more, and see how the months vary.

In addition to taking your temperature, take notes on your cervical mucus. This is a sure indication of when you are ovulating, so it lets you know if your temperature readings are off by a few days. You may also ovulate and have too little mucus for the sperm to swim through in order to conceive. There are different methods on how to check exactly. The easiest way is to wipe the vaginal area with toilet paper before you urinate or make a bowel movement. It is also a good idea to check again after you use the bathroom to see if any mucus has made its way out. Each day that you take your temperature, note what the mucus was overall for the day, too. You will most likely notice this easily.

Obviously when you have your period, you will make note of that. After your period you will most likely be dry (have no mucus) for a few days. Then, as the cycle progresses, you will have a little mucus (described as similar to the coating on sticky rice), followed by a lot of mucus (similar to an egg white consistency) leading up to the big ovulation day. The more mucus, the more fertile your body is. After ovulation, your mucus will become sticky again or dry up. You will then get a period or a positive pregnancy test.

Using both thermometer readings and mucus assessments are inexpensive and relatively easy to do. You can also buy an ovulation predictor kit online or at the drug store as a back-up method. The issue with relying solely on test kits is that they cannot detect if your temperatures or hormonal levels are off, or if you have the proper amount of cervical mucus. When trying to conceive, if you show your chart to a qualified professional, he or she can help you detect potential hidden issues. Some such issues could be hormonal. For instance, you might have low progesterone levels if your temperature doesn't elevate after ovulation. You could also have a luteal phase defect if you ovulate very late in the cycle. This is why I emphasize the importance of charting rather than just using an ovulation predictor kit.

Also, you might receive an inaccurate reading on an ovulation predictor kit if you have a difficult time holding urine for four hours during the day. Drinking lots of fluids during the day may also dilute the urine enough to make the kit unable to detect the ovulation surge. If I had solely relied on such a kit, I might have missed my window with my recent baby. Since I knew my temperature and mucus levels, I said to my husband, "The time is *now*!"

Most kits say to test the first day's urine, but in some cases, your LH surge may happen in the afternoon. This means that you may miss that window of ovulation—like I almost did—if you rely on the kit alone. The following morning your temperature may spike and you would have already ovulated. Again this is why timing and knowing when you ovulate is crucial. This is especially true for people who are extremely busy, working different schedules, traveling for business, or what have you. If your mate is away at sea, there will be no baby! Here is the best advice if you want to use the kits in addition to basal body temperature charting and checking your cervical mucus. As you get close to ovulation and see the signs of egg white mucus, start testing with the kits twice a day in case you have an afternoon or evening surge.

Boost Your Chances

Also around the time of ovulation, you may increase your chances of implantation if you eat pineapple, specifically the core. Chinese Medicine has found it helpful with natural conception and IVF.[25] There is an enzyme called Bromelain in pineapple, which is thought to help ensure successful embryonic implantation. It can increase blood to the uterus and act as a blood thinner. For women experiencing miscarriages due to positive phospholipid antibodies, this tip might be especially useful. Bromelain also has anti-inflammatory properties. Advice varies since there are no known studies that are conclusive. I suggest you start by eating one to two fresh pineapple slices with the core the day of ovulation/IVF or after for about a week or longer. Eating it too soon, though, can affect cervical mucus acidity. Eating too much can also be bad for the pregnancy—some cultures even use it to end pregnancy or start labor. It is best to not eat pineapple during the beginning stages of pregnancy either because it thins blood. There is also some information out there on eating Brazil Nuts around the time of ovulation, about five nuts per day.[26] They can help thicken the lining of the uterus and be good for sperm health and testosterone levels. Brazil nuts are said to help boost selenium and are high in zinc.[27] It is worth a try for both you and your partner to eat a few Brazil nuts as a snack!

Now that you know how to combine a diet and timing for conception, the waiting game begins. In the days leading up to either a positive pregnancy test or another period, you may want to take extra care of yourself. This time can be bliss or stressful for a couple wanting to conceive. The days of waiting can seem like forever. One of the best things to do is to take your mind off of it (which is not easy), and try to relax! Avoid stress. If you are practicing gentle yoga, meditation, or prayer, now would be a good time to do those things! You also want to avoid all toxins and stressors.

Because you might be eating for two, now is a really important time to watch your diet. If you are predisposed for diabetes, have pre-diabetes, or are sensitive to blood sugar fluctuations, for instance, now is also a very good time to avoid sugar. According to research, if you have diabetes or are borderline diabetic, irregular insulin could cause complications and even miscarriage.[28] Try to be positive, and if it doesn't happen this month, it eventually will happen! Have faith!

CHAPTER NINE: FERTILITY MASSAGE, ACUPUNCTURE, REIKI, AND YOGA

Relaxation is very important when trying to encourage and support fertility. Fertility massage, acupuncture, Reiki, and yoga are several excellent methods that promote relaxation, and some also support fertility. Most are done with the help of a professional, while yoga can be easily done on your own or with an instructor. You can use any one of these methods—or a combination of several—to help make you more apt to conceive.

Fertility Massage

You have probably heard (or experienced) how wonderful it can be to get a massage for physical aches and pains, especially during pregnancy. But have you ever heard of a fertility massage? A fertility massage is intended to get your body primed for conception. It helps to warm the uterus and belly, which is key to conception in Chinese medicine. "Warm belly to hold a warm baby" is how I like to think of it.

Cultures ranging from South America to China and India focus on the abdomen as a place of healing. Three of the six chakras are also located in the abdomen: Mooladhara, Swadhisthana, and Manipura. When trying to conceive, you want to have chi flowing freely throughout your body, as opposed to having chi that is blocked or stagnant. When chi flows freely, the body is more able to heal itself and to keep processes—like those involved in conception—functioning optimally.

Because stagnation or blockages are not good for fertility or conception, I recommend fertility massage. Fertility massage can help by getting blood to flow freely to the abdomen. During the massage, nutrient-rich blood is sent to your reproductive organs, and if it passes unhindered through the abdomen, it can restore these organs and help clear out toxins. Specific treatments are needed to heal certain issues. For example, we tend to hold our emotions in the abdomen, so being able to free the abdomen and reproductive organs of stressful emotions may be necessary when you are trying to conceive.

There are many types of fertility massages from which to choose. Depending on where you live, you can find massage therapists in your area who are trained at doing fertility massages and I will explain some of them now.

- Arvigo Maya abdominal massage (www.arvigotherapy.com)is an adaptation of Mayan healing techniques. Dr. Rosita Arvigo, whose specialty is in realigning connective tissue, developed it. Arvigo spent ten years living in the rainforest region of Belize as an apprentice to Don Elijio Panti, who was known as the "last Mayan master healer" upon his death at 103 years of age.

  In the 1990s, Arvigo began teaching others her own method of abdominal massage—techniques she had adapted while studying with Panti. Arvigo was a proponent of the Mayan medicine tenet that one must show gratitude for the plants, given by God (the Divine) for their healing properties, for protecting and prolonging life. This was an integral part of her teachings with students in workshops and spiritual intensives.

- Self-Fertility Massage, which women do on themselves, is based on the Asian organ massage known as *Chi Nei Tsang*, as well as acupressure and deep tissue massage.

  To begin, lie down comfortably and take a few deep breaths to relax. Begin by pressing the tips of your fingers near your belly button. Then massage while spiraling outward away from the belly button in a clockwise circular motion, moving farther and farther away from your belly button. Continue for about fifteen minutes. Do not do a self-fertility massage when you have your period or once you ovulate.

Hethir Rodriguez, who is an expert on Self-Fertility Massage, also recommends massaging the middle of the bottom of the big toe, which affects the pituitary gland and in turn helps maintain hormonal balance. She says to press firmly and massage in a circular motion. She recommends doing the massage daily after your period up until you ovulate. If you have other reproductive issues such as PCOS, scar tissues, blocked tubes, cysts, endometriosis, or a tilted uterus, you may benefit from this kind of massage. As circulation is improved to the abdomen, it can improve your digestive and reproductive systems, too.

• Mercier Therapy, created by Dr. Jennifer Mercier in 2005, is a deep, visceral manual massage of the abdomen. Mercier trained as a midwife and has a PhD in Natural Medicine. In Mercier Therapy, the practitioner feels the uterus, fallopian tubes, and ovaries to make sure they are movable and not stiff. This can free up the organs and restores blood flow. Not only did Dr. Mercier create her own form of fertility massage, she enlisted her students to perform the massage on her. Mercier wanted to get pregnant after suffering from endometriosis and being told she would need IVF.

Mercier is the author of *Women's Optimal Pelvic Health with Mercier Therapy* in 2010. She recently completed a four-year study on the Mercier Therapy method, and is releasing the documentary *Fertility* about her work. Patients who follow her protocol have an 83% success rate. Most of the patients she has had success with have had endometriosis, PCOS, or thyroid issues. This protocol includes six one-hour sessions of abdominal work.

There are thirty-five therapists in the United States trained in her therapy. Visit www.merciertherapy.com to find a practitioner listing or you can visit Dr. Mercier in the Chicago area for a weekend of treatment.

One way to tell if you have stagnation, or even a tilted uterus, is if you have brown blood during your period. This means you have old blood. Surprisingly, many women have a tilted or displaced uterus, and do not even know it. This can be due to a fall, car accident, horseback riding, running, gymnastics or other high impact sports, chronic constipation, overstretching from a previous pregnancy, or even something as common as wearing high heels. Who knew?

Unfortunately, a lot of women are told by their OB-GYN that a tilted uterus is not a big deal. They are being misled, because having a tilted uterus can affect your ability to conceive. "When the uterus is incorrectly aligned, the normal flow of blood and lymph are constricted and can disrupt nerve connection. The circulation of blood to the uterus, ovaries, bladder, and bowel is blocked."[29] According to the Maya, a woman's center is her uterus. "If a woman's uterus is out of balance, so is she," says Don Elijio Panti.[30] Fertility massage can help reposition your uterus and clear stagnation.

Fertility massage is also helpful if you have painful periods. A lot of women do and think it is just a monthly fact. Periods really should not be painful. Imagine how many women are walking around every month with mild cramps or ones so severely debilitating that they cannot even get out of bed? Ladies, this is not normal. Instead of popping a pill, go get or give yourself a massage. Rather than the traditional approach of prescribing birth control pills, which is obviously not the correct option if you're trying to conceive, consult with a massage professional who can guide you through alternative methods.

The fertility massage will usually correct issues in roughly one to three months, depending on how severe the issue.[31]

Acupuncture

While alternative treatments like fertility massage may be less well known, acupuncture is something that most of us have heard of—and maybe even tried. In use for almost three thousand years, acupuncture is one of the oldest healing practices in the world. According to Traditional Chinese Medicine, acupuncture stimulates specific acupressure points, of which there are 350 in the body. By doing so it corrects any imbalances or blockages of chi through channels in the body known as meridians. Acupuncture can treat various ailments, and it is especially helpful for preparing the body for conception if you have underlying fertility issues.

Many acupuncturists are also trained in herbal medicine, and many specialize in fertility issues. If you choose to use acupuncture to help enhance fertility, you will go once or twice a week. Sometimes the acupuncturist will combine different herbs for different times in your cycle. A chart of your cycle will also be helpful to give the acupuncturist so he or she will know your basal body temperatures and detect any possible hormonal imbalances.

Unlike most other medical practitioners, acupuncturists will look at your tongue when examining you. Because they are taught to diagnose medical issues this way, an acupuncturist will look at the tongue closely for shape, color, and coating which gives them clues as to what is happening throughout the body. For example, a pale tongue can indicate anemia—and detect stagnation or dehydration. As part of the exam, acupuncturists typically take your pulse at the wrist to feel how strong the blood is flowing.

After a brief exam is done, the acupuncturist will begin to treat you with needles. You disrobe as necessary, and usually lie on a table during treatment. Needles are then placed in different parts of the body, from the head to the feet. Some may be placed in the abdomen, depending on where you are in your cycle. You may feel the needle being inserted if the area is tight, sore, or needs attention for another reason. Don't worry— after the needle has been in place for a few seconds, any uncomfortable sensation will lessen.

After all of the appropriate needles are placed in the body, you will relax for a bit. These needles redirect the energy in the body, allowing the chi to flow smoothly, which often helps with conception. Besides calming the body and mind, acupuncture treatments open pathways in ways that we do not understand.

Even for those receiving IVF treatments, it has been known to help with implantation.

Acupuncture can also be used to induce labor. While most doctors induce with Pitocin, a procedure that can put stress on mother and child, acupuncturists are able to induce in a more natural, gentle manner. There are many reasons to induce labor, which you can discuss with your practitioner. If you are getting pressure to induce, and you are at or past your due date, acupuncture is a wonderful option. There are certain pressure points—in the tops of your shoulders, at the lower inner side of your lower leg, and at the point between your thumb and pointer finger—which are known to stimulate labor. For maximum effect, go to an acupuncturist. You can also use pressure points on your own to induce or ease labor.

- The point known as **Spleen 6** (inner side of lower leg) can reduce discomfort, shorten labor according to a study at the University of North Carolina, encourage labor by strengthening contractions that are weak, and aid in the ripening of the cervix.[32] We used Spleen 6 when in the hospital during our first birth and could see the effect the pressure was having on my labor when we looked at the monitors. That made me a believer for sure!
- **Bladder 60** (between the Achilles tendon and the ankle) is a great point if your baby has not "dropped" yet.
- **Bladder 67** (on your little toe) is good if you have a breech baby who needs help turning. This should be done well before the due date if the baby is breech. Bladder 67 is also generally good for inducing labor.
- **Kidney 1** (located on the bottom of the foot) is thought to help calm women during labor.
- **Large Intestine 4** (between the pointer finger and thumb) is an excellent point to induce labor, and will also help with headaches, toothaches, or discomfort in the head. About the size of a nickel, it's easy to find for most people and it's very popular for managing pain and making contractions more efficient.
- **Gallbladder 21** (on the top of the shoulder, directly above the nipple) can stimulate contractions, help baby descend, and assist

in releasing a retained placenta when all or part of the placenta has not been delivered in the third stage of labor. Although rare and more common in pre-term labors, this can increase the risk of bleeding if the placenta is not delivered in an hour after the birth. Along with pressure point stimulation, breastfeeding will also help by releasing the hormone oxytocin.

- **Bladder 32** (midway between the dimple in the sacrum and the spine) is great for ripening and dilating the cervix. A lot of women have found that it can also provide a numbing effect when pressure is applied during contractions.

- **Gall bladder 29** (The hip point is located horizontally from the top of the crease of the buttock near the hipbone.) This point can help move labor along during transition or during a contraction.

Acupuncture is very beneficial to your health during all phases of pregnancy. If you have never tried it or simply have a fear of needles, it is worth a shot, no pun intended. I am now a big fan of acupuncture after overcoming my fear of needles. I used to pass out when getting blood drawn! This is a completely different experience. The needles are superfine, and sometimes you do not even feel them. I used acupuncture before all of my pregnancies and believe it, along with some dietary changes, helped my ability to conceive. Used in the first trimester, it lessened the nausea from morning sickness, too. It is a good natural option for whatever ails you in pregnancy. I even used it to help induce one of my labors! Try acupuncture and see how it makes you feel.

Reiki

If you are familiar with alternative treatments, you may have heard of Reiki. Catalina Rivera, a Reiki Master, explained to me: "Reiki is a Japanese technique for deep relaxation, wellbeing, healing, and personal growth. Through energy work and gentle touch, the recipient is immersed in a deep state of relaxation that promotes and strengthens his or her innate capacity for healing, harmony, and insight."

Reiki was developed over a hundred years ago by Dr. Mikao Usui of Japan, and made its way to the United States in the 1960s. Usually performed by a Reiki practitioner, you can even learn to heal yourself with Reiki. A simple explanation is that hands are placed on or just above the body in various positions to move chi (energy) to facilitate healing. He described Reiki poetically:

Catalina says, "The beauty of Reiki is that it is a gentle and effective process. No lengthy conversations or analysis required. What is no longer serving you is released, and insight comes naturally where needed. Your inner wisdom is activated, and you begin to make better decisions for yourself and your life. Best of all, there are no side effects or contraindications—it works synergistically with everything else you may be doing for your health and wellbeing. Plus, it is safe in pregnancy and all stages of life."

This is what Catalina Rivera has to say on Reiki and conception "As most of us are aware—to some degree—it is the interplay of our body, emotions, mind and spirit that dictate our reality. When trying to conceive attention to our whole being is crucial, even more so when things are not going as smoothly as desired. Reiki is a wonderful holistic tool to round off the more commonly used methods to enhance fertility and adds elements that most people don't address or aren't sure how to."

I received my first Reiki session from Catalina, who studied Reiki in Santiago, Chile and had been practicing for thirteen years. Catalina is also a labor and delivery nurse who has used Reiki with laboring mothers. I wasn't sure what to expect at the session, so I lay on the table, relaxed in my comfortable clothing, and kept my eyes closed, ready to accept any and all healing. I was in the process of weaning my daughter off of breastfeeding in hopes of conceiving another child. As Catalina placed her hands over me, I felt a sensation of both warmth and energy at the same time. I grew more and more relaxed throughout the session and even fell asleep.

When I awoke, I was alert, clearheaded, and deeply relaxed. I didn't seek treatment for any physical ailments or medical issues, so my body felt the same after the treatment. What was different was an overwhelming feeling of calm and good. Your experience will be unique to you, although others have reported an experience similar to mine. This overall sense of well-being lasted for a couple of days, and I conceived another baby a couple months later!

Reiki can be very helpful when trying to conceive. It can help balance hormones, strengthen organs, and counteract stress and its tremendous impact on our health. (Reiki is even used in many hospitals now for cancer and pain management, too.) Finally, and most importantly in many cases, it can help you release any lingering emotional baggage or present-day fears, conscious or unconscious, which may be affecting your fertility. By supporting emotional and mental health, treatments can help you get into the "Mommy Mindset" before you decide to conceive. Positive thinking and positive energy are essential when trying to conceive, and Reiki promotes this naturally.

In the same way that acupuncture gets chi (energy) flowing with the use of needles, Reiki can restore any energy that may be lacking or blocked. Because Reiki focuses on improving the health of your chakras, a practitioner will pay particular attention to your first and second chakras if there are blockages in the reproductive area. The first chakra, or root chakra, relates to procreation and birth. It has the symbol of the lotus. The second chakra, the sacral chakra, is associated with the reproductive system. Its symbol is the crescent moon, which represents femininity in the womb. Stimulating these areas during Reiki may be all you need to set you on your reproductive path. There is even a case study of a woman who had PCOS and conceived after four months of Reiki treatment. She was so impacted by Reiki that she became a Reiki master herself![33]

It may take a few sessions to restore balance and replenish energy. It depends on each person's overall physical and mental health, and energy level when beginning treatments. Reiki encourages the entire conception process and "can be used throughout a woman's cycle to support the growth of follicles and recruitment of healthy eggs, the fertilization of eggs, and assisting the embryo to implant in the uterine lining."[34]

Once you are pregnant, Reiki can help reduce nausea and exhaustion in the first trimester; it also helps reduce sleep problems, anxiety, and a variety of other conditions. During my last weeks of pregnancy, it left me feeling wonderful, and relieved the anxiety I had over all my preparations for the third baby. Used during labor, it can alleviate discomfort in a laboring mother. Reiki performed by doctors and nurses in a woman's hospital in the Czech Republic had laboring mothers more in control and relaxed during their birthing experiences, and their labors were easier overall.[35]

I would highly recommend trying Reiki and learning how Reiki treatments make you feel. It is completely safe during pre-conception, pregnancy, and during labor. If you are looking for an alternative treatment, Reiki is definitely worth exploring.

Yoga

Yoga is thousands of years old and has evolved into many different types, including Hatha, Vinyasa, Bikram, Ashtanga, Power, Kundalini, Kripalu, and Yin. It is a great practice to start, if you are not already familiar with it. If you begin practicing yoga before your pregnancy, you will be ahead of the game if you decide to join a prenatal yoga class, too. This will allow you to be able to relax more thoroughly instead of being worried about learning the poses. Yoga can lower blood pressure, and increase the strength and flexibility needed for pregnancy and birth. By connecting your breath to your body and quieting your mind, yoga will prime you for pregnancy. You will gain focus and calm, improve sleep and reduce stress.

Depending on the type you choose, yoga can be practiced before and during pregnancy with some modifications. During pregnancy, the safest types are prenatal yoga and Hatha yoga. Continuing your practice during pregnancy will help keep your muscles flexible and strong when it comes time to give birth, and help reduce or eliminate back pain, nausea, headaches, and shortness of breath. According to the Mayo Clinic, it may even reduce the risk of preterm labor, pregnancy-induced hypertension, and intrauterine restriction.[36]

Hatha yoga is the foundation of many different yoga styles. Because Hatha focuses on the basic poses, breathing, and some meditation techniques, it is a great style for beginners to learn. Although it can be done throughout pregnancy, it is best to let a qualified teacher guide you as to which poses are safe to do during pregnancy, which should be modified, and which should be avoided. For example, yoga poses that should be avoided during pregnancy include those where you are lying on your back or belly, backward or forward bends, and twisting poses, since they may put pressure on your abdomen. As pregnancy progresses, listen to your body during yoga and do not overexert yourself. As with any exercise, it is important to stay well-hydrated and not overheat. By practicing early in pregnancy, or starting even before you conceive, you are more likely to approach your practice with confidence and to experience deep relaxation, which is so helpful when you reach the later stages of your pregnancy.

Prenatal yoga poses are poses adapted for pregnant mothers. They are safe exercises to do throughout pregnancy, and can help keep your core and pelvic floor muscles strong as your growing baby pulls your body in all sorts of directions. Having a strong body can aid in an easier delivery, which is good news for first time moms!

If you have taken a few classes and have a good idea how to do the poses, you can purchase yoga videos to do at home. This can be a great way to wind down from a long day. I especially enjoy *Shiva Rea's Prenatal Yoga* video, as it shows three different women in various stages and levels. This type of program will give you an idea of how to modify your yoga practice throughout your pregnancy.

It is good to have your own yoga mat, a block or a strap to use during yoga, and sometimes a blanket. You can find a variety of yoga accessories online. If you are not interested in doing a yoga video, look for a prenatal yoga class. It will feel good to join with other mothers-to-be, plus you will enjoy feeling calm and centered while you are pregnant.

Fertility massage, acupuncture, Reiki, and yoga can have a huge impact on your health and wellbeing. Being open to other alternative options is something women sometimes use as a last resort. My suggestion is to incorporate any or all of these long before that! You can relax and recharge with these safe and natural methods. By incorporating one or more of them into your pre-pregnancy plan, you just may have an easier time conceiving.

CHAPTER TEN: GESTATIONAL DIABETES AND NATURAL BIRTH OPTIONS

Once you have a positive pregnancy test, you say, "Now What?" First of all, congratulations on a job well done! The next few months can go by very quickly. Enjoy them! But don't go back to old habits and food choices. The journey to healthy living is critical during pregnancy. You are what you eat, breath in, and live around—these will all influence your baby. Maybe you did a few "Green" changes and would like to begin to transform your life and home into the ultimate environment to bring your new baby into. Yay, you! Now is the time to nest and take whatever steps you like to continue "Going Green" now that you have conceived. Again, do not let it overwhelm you. Keep stress to a minimum. Do steps day-by-day or week-by-week.

In this chapter I discuss gestational diabetes, how to naturally induce, drug-free birth options, perineal massage, and delaying the umbilical cord cutting. This knowledge will arm you with the tools to design a stress-free delivery. Also, putting your team of knowledgeable professionals in place now is a great idea. When you need support for breastfeeding, babywearing, mom groups, etc, you will not feel so lost when you need help.

Gestational Diabetes

There will be things that come up during pregnancy that you can control with alternative therapies mentioned earlier. As you go through pregnancy, you will encounter many tests. One of these tests you for gestational diabetes around 24 to 28 weeks of pregnancy. Gestational diabetes is a type of diabetes women can get during pregnancy. If you are overweight before your pregnancy, if you are over 35 years old, or if you have a family history of diabetes, you may have a greater risk. The glucose drink you are given at the test contains a solution that is not organic and contains harmful food coloring. There are some midwives who allow you to substitute a meal for the glucose drink. However, if you are already at risk for gestational diabetes, this may not be an option for you.

With gestational diabetes, you may have abnormally high blood sugar levels when you wake up in the morning or an hour after you have a meal. If your blood sugar levels are too high, it can affect the baby and make his blood sugar levels rise as well. There is also something known as dawn phenomenon which could be causing your levels to rise in the morning as well. You can learn more on this in the book written by G. E. Frazier entitled *The Dawn Phenomenon*. In many cases drugs may not be needed and diet alone will control your diabetes. The drugs prescribed may not be entirely safe during pregnancy. Read the ingredients and see for yourself. I can personally attest to having a severe reaction to insulin after being persuaded to try insulin before bed in order to get my morning number down. They were only in the 90s but the endocrinologist insisted it was too high for my second pregnancy. Right after my husband injected me, I shook all over and it wasn't from my sugar levels since I tested them while still shaking! I believe it was the ingredients my body was rejecting that were not safe. Luckily I stopped shaking after drinking lots of water and did not need to go to the emergency room. I was able to control my levels the remainder of the pregnancy without drugs and the baby was fine. Makes me wonder if I really had it at all.

In a lot of cases, you can control gestational diabetes by diet and by getting proper amounts sleep. Sleep can do wonders to heal the body! If you are diagnosed, you will need to see a nutritionist to learn how to eat properly and keep your blood sugar under control. If you already were eliminating sugar prior to pregnancy, you will probably already be on a pretty healthy diet. Sometimes, though, things just happen during pregnancy. Try to roll with it. Other than diet, I found a few helpful tips to avoid medication when controlling blood sugar levels.

To start, apple cider vinegar has been helpful in lowering blood sugar levels. A quick option is to make a refreshing drink. I suggest my Apple Cider Drink.

Apple Cider Drink

- 2-3 teaspoons Bragg's Apple Cider Vinegar
- 3 drops of Young Living Essential Orange Oil
- Fill the Glass with Filtered Water
- Add Stevia (Green Powdered Preferred)

Stir and add ice if you like. Enjoy!

I personally used this drink during my third pregnancy at least every other day. If I ate a meal with ingredients that could spike my blood sugar—something high in carbs such as corn or gluten-free bread—I drank it more often.

Sleep also had an impact on my fasting blood sugar levels in the morning. If I slept at least eight hours, my blood sugar level was below 90. If I got less than eight hours, my blood sugar level was between 90-96. While that is not alarming, it is over the recommended number for a morning blood sugar, which is below 90.

Some find it helpful to take Young Living Ocotea Essential Oil. This oil is indigenous to South America and is useful in maintaining normal blood sugar levels. Some people take it before meals in a capsule form, while others add it to boiling water and sip it before a meal. I prefer putting a few drops in a spoonful of coconut oil.

While these tips will not work for everyone, you can try them. Please speak to a medical professional if you need further help regulating your gestational diabetes.

Inducing Naturally

Another bump in the road if you have gestational diabetes, other health issues, or if the baby simply just does not want to come after you have reached the 41st or 42nd week of pregnancy, is the talk of "inducing" or "induction." Being Green means inducing while still following an all-natural birth protocol as opposed to starting labor by introducing chemicals into the mother's system, which most hospitals rely on. Luckily, there are several things you can do to naturally get your body into labor.

- **Sex**—The prostaglandins in the sperm can help you begin labor, thin, and dilate your cervix, and orgasms produce Ocytoxin (the natural kind) and can start contractions.
- **Spicy foods**—This works for some women, others say it just causes a trip to the bathroom.
- **Eggplant Parmesan**—Something in the eggplant works, maybe the spices?
- **Pineapple**—Contain the enzyme Bromelain, which can soften the cervix, bring on muscle contractions, and possibly reduce labor time.
- **Evening Primrose Oil Capsules**—Inserted vaginally can help the cervix thin and dilate. Do not take if you have placenta previa, and speak to your midwife before using.
- **Red Raspberry Leaf tea**—Contained in some pregnancy teas as part of the blend, by itself may induce labor.
- **Castor oil**—Taken to get your bowels moving which, in turn, can start labor. Note: Use with caution. Some say it can be a rough process and that it can lead to dehydration.
- **Walking**—Walking, or walking up and down stairs or escalators in a mall.
- **Acupuncture**—Inserting needles in the proper points will move the baby down and get contractions going. More than one session or the use of electrical needle stimulation may be needed as well.

- **Acupressure**—Applying pressure with your hands or fingers into the proper points in the body that you would with acupuncture.
- **Essential Oils**—Young Living Clary Sage and Jasmine. Note: Use with caution. According to some professionals, these may only work if labor is near or already started. From personal experience, I used Young Living Clary Sage aromatically a few times the day before I went into labor. The day labor started I applied Clary Sage to the pressure points on the hand, lower leg, and shoulders and labor started a few hours later.

Natural, Drug-Free Birth Options

Choosing a birth plan is a very personal decision. Some women know without a doubt that they do not want any drugs, while others have a very low threshold for pain and will gladly take whatever relief they can get. A lot of the pain or discomfort during labor comes from fear. Fear can especially worsen pain should you not have coping techniques. That said, having the proper tools to enable you to birth naturally makes a big difference in your confidence level. The mind over matter concept can play a key role in achieving a natural birth. Also, having an OB-GYN or Midwife onboard who knows your desires will help in this as well.

You will also want to decide who you want to be present at your birth. Some couples want the entire family in the room while others just want it to be them and the doula, midwife and nurses or other professionals. Some couples decide a home birth is a safe option for them and prepare with their midwife to make that possible. Think about who makes you calm and peaceful and who stresses you out. Carefully choosing your team to have in the room will make all the difference as it will set the tone and energy during birth. The calmer the better!

We have all heard of women who did not even know they were pregnant or did not know they were in labor until a baby descended. (Many gave birth in the bathroom!) While these births give us all hope of a pain-free, natural birth, often labor can take quite a while to progress, especially if you are giving birth to your first child. Learning from an experienced teacher is a great way to prepare. While we never truly know what to expect, a class will give you a better understanding of what might happen and teach you some tools for coping if something unexpected occurs during your labor.

The Bradley Method

It is a good idea to take a natural birthing class like a Bradley Method* class. This is also known as husband-coached birthing. In their own words: "The Bradley Method* teaches natural childbirth and views birth as a natural process. It is our belief that most women with proper education, preparation, and the help of a loving and supportive coach can be taught to give birth naturally. The Bradley Method* is a system of natural labor techniques in which a woman and her coach play an active part. It is a simple method of increasing self-awareness, teaching a woman how to deal with the stress of labor by tuning in to her own body. The Bradley Method* encourages mothers to trust their bodies using natural breathing, relaxation, nutrition, exercise, and education."[37]

I especially like that you are taught the stages of birth and comfortable birthing positions with this method. Most women think they have to stay in a hospital bed, surprisingly they do not!

Mongan Hypnobirthing

I also loved my Hypnobirthing class, which my husband actually found for us only a month and a half before I gave birth to our first child! In their own words: "Mongan Method HypnoBirthing® is a simple, straightforward program, thoughtfully developed over the years to remind mothers of the simplicity of birth itself. Just as the majority of birthing women do not need interventions and procedures for safe and healthy birth, they do not need a complex set of exercises and scripts to prepare themselves for peaceful, calm, and comfortable birthing. The birthing body and the baby know just what to do. Mongan Method HypnoBirthing® is designed to teach women to trust in Nature's way of birth, and to relax and let their bodies do what is needed. By practicing a few key techniques, mothers program their minds and condition their bodies to birth easily. When it comes to programming and conditioning, variety is not necessarily a good thing. Repetition is what gets the best result."[38]

By listening to various CD's from a Mongan HypnoBirthing teacher during the weeks leading up to my delivery, I learned relaxation techniques and gained confidence to birth naturally and drug free with my second and third births. I prepped for each birth with my Hypnobirthing CD's and feel they made all the difference.

Sometimes problems arise during labor, which require our midwives, doulas, or doctors to perform an emergency C-section. If surgery becomes your only option, then relaxation techniques will help. Know, however, that an epidural will greatly increase your chance of intervention (with drugs or surgery). This said, if you prep for a natural, drug-free birth, you are more likely to have a natural, vaginal birth.

Doula Support

Another major stress-reliever during birth is having a doula. Doulas are trained to support women during labor, delivery, and just after the birth. The word doula in Greek means "a woman who serves." They offer continuous emotional and physical support during this amazing experience. Some may massage or apply pressure to your back to help comfort you. Mothers find that births attended by doulas are usually shorter and less stressful.[39]

They help calm you and inform you of what is going on during your birth. Having this calm stream of information sometimes is all women need to feel cared for while delivering their baby. Doulas can also assist with breastfeeding as soon as your baby is born. Having them there to help the baby get latched on to your breast properly is a comforting start for mother and child.

Although you have a nine to ten month relationship with your midwife or OBGYN, unfortunately, they may not be the one to deliver the baby—a likelihood that is not conveyed to many expecting moms.

In fact, depending on the practitioner, your midwife or doctor may only rarely be in the room to support you during your labor. In contrast, your doula will be there with you every step of the way. This is why it is crucial to have your partner take birthing classes with you and for you both to choose a doula who you both connect with. This will ensure that you feel incredibly supported during delivery. Also, be sure the doula is not overbooked with other pending births. If you are truly counting on one particular person, and she has to attend another birth when you go into labor, she might send someone in her place who you may have only met once.

You also may choose to hire a postpartum doula to help once you have delivered the baby. These doulas will help with newborn care, family adjustment, meal preparation, and light household cleanup. They are not to be confused with a baby nurse, who focuses only on the baby. Postpartum doulas also offer support, companionship, and education during this transitional time of becoming new parents. They may be especially valuable if your partner has a very limited time off from work or if you live far away from family or friends.

Some couples feel they need space and need to go it alone, while others welcome support of any form. This is a personal decision. There are options and there is no right or wrong way—only whatever feels right for your new family.

Perineal Massage

One of the most valuable things I have ever learned about prepping for birth is perineal massage or stretching. I learned about perineal massage during my hypnobirthing class before the birth of my first child. It involves stretching the area between the vagina and the anus, otherwise known as the perineum. This is the area that stretches during a vaginal childbirth. Using this technique can help you avoid tearing or cutting, and, hopefully, the need for stitches. You can do a perineal massage alone or with the help of your partner.

By performing daily perineal massage weeks prior to the birth, you will prepare the perineum for the stretching that will occur during birth. You might wonder, is this really necessary? Any woman who has a birth-related tear will tell you that it is not comfortable having stitches in the perineal area. Granted, a small tear is better than a large C-section incision, but not having any tear at all is the best outcome and is totally possible!

So how do you perform this perineal massage/stretch? First, get comfortable. Some potential ways to perform a solo massage are:

- 33-34 weeks in pregnancy. Position yourself on a bed propped up with pillows. Stand in the shower with a foot on a stool or sit on a shower seat (being careful not to fall over). You can also get comfortable on a toilet either standing with a foot on the toilet to secure your balance or sitting on the toilet edge. Start with a lubricant, such as organic olive oil. You can add a drop of Young Living Frankincense to the oil, which will help protect the delicate tissue during stretching.

  Next, insert one or two thumbs about an inch into the vagina. Slowly and delicately push down toward your anus. Keep your thumbs in this position so you feel a slight stretching sensation. Do not push too hard in the beginning or you could accidentally tear.

  Next, slowly massage the lower half of your vagina in a U-shaped movement. You can continue the process of massage and stretching for about ten minutes. This is a slow, gradual process and will take some time to get your perineum stretched to allow for the birth of the baby.

- As your pregnancy progresses. If you are having trouble feeling a stretch or reaching around your large belly, for instance, it might be time for your partner to help you achieve a full stretch. After all, didn't he take part in this baby making process? Start by getting in a comfortable position where your partner can reach your vagina with his index fingers. *Note: This is not the same as solo instructions, where I advised you to use your thumbs.* Using organic olive oil, have your partner insert his fingers about an inch and begin pressing down toward your anus until you feel a slight stretching sensation. Be sure to communicate with your partner to let him know when to stop pushing so you do not tear. Once you feel stretched, have him massage the bottom of your vagina in a U-shaped motion.

Doing this massage with your partner may feel awkward at first, but it can turn into a relaxing nightly ritual before bed or even foreplay! In this way you are prepping for the baby to descend easily and minimizing discomfort during birth. It also can become a quiet bonding time between you and your partner as you prepare in the very last weeks before the baby arrives. Ten minutes before bed, or whenever your schedule allows, is all it takes, and it truly can prevent tears.

After a week or so of solo or partner-assisted massage, you will notice your perineum has more elasticity. This will allow the head of the baby to move more easily through the vagina and hopefully minimize or prevent tearing of the perineum.

Another word of advice for anyone reading this and prepping for a second child; Do the massage even if this is not your first baby. After a first birth, the tissues of the vagina and perineum will eventually lose elasticity and go back to the way they were before. In some cases, the vagina and perineum become even tighter. I have known women who tore worse with their second babies, probably because they did not do perineal massage in their second pregnancy. Some of them thought, "I already had a baby it should be easier." Though the labor length itself may be much shorter, the skin still needs prepping to stretch. When you train for your second marathon, do you train fewer hours or put in less commitment? No. You are looking for better results, so you train just as hard, if not harder! Going from one tiny stitch from your first birth to no tearing or stitching is something we should all wish to achieve with our births—not to mention this makes getting around after birth much easier on the mother. You will not require ice or a donut-shaped pillow to sit on while you cuddle your little one for the first time. Also, this makes the ride home from the hospital a pleasurable one. Potholes and vaginal stitches do not mix well.

By prepping the perineum, you are doing yourself a great service in preventing painful tears and alleviating pressure that the baby's head causes during crowning. If perineal massage can alleviate swelling, tearing, and discomfort, go for it!

Delay Cord Cutting

Once the baby has popped out, hopefully easily, I suggest that you delay cutting the cord. Research indicates that it is best to place the baby on the mother's chest or abdomen and let the pulsating of the umbilical cord continue for a few minutes. As we are now learning, delaying the cord cutting until the cord stops pulsating is most helpful to get more blood to the baby upon birth. This gives the baby more iron and higher hemoglobin, which helps prevent anemia.[40] Most doctors are quick to cut the cord as soon as the baby is delivered. This is a mistake. Ask your doctor or midwife to wait until you've stopped pulsating.

Another benefit of delayed cord cutting, according to one study in Mexico, is that it may help protect your baby from lead poisoning.[41] The logic is that having low-iron can make the body more susceptible to absorbing lead. Even if you add iron to your diet for up to six months after birth, this still might not give your baby as much iron as he would have had if the cord wasn't cut right away. One reason why you may not be able to delay cord cutting is if the baby was born in distress and needs immediate medical attention. Also, if you are planning on Cord Blood Registry, your doctor or midwife may need to cut a little sooner as well to get the blood to storage.

Whatever birth plan you decide on, know that the most important thing is that the baby arrives safely. These tips can help you have a successful, healthy pregnancy and delivery. Good luck!

CHAPTER ELEVEN: ESSENTIAL OILS FOR PREGNANCY AND BIRTH

Though essential oils have been around for centuries, they are only now gaining popularity for all sorts of uses. Some people use them as aromatherapy, which means they diffuse them into the air, to aid with prayer, meditation, and/or relaxation. Others use them topically or internally to support health in various ways. Quality oils like Young Living are far superior to others: If you do not know where they are sourced and how they are grown, it can be like eating pesticide-laden foods. This is especially important when you are priming your body for pregnancy.

Essential oils are a great natural way to support your health and can prep your body and mind for an ideal pregnancy. As always, listen to your body and run anything by your doctor if you have a health condition. Like food and fragrances, some essential oils may not work for all people. You will have your favorites and ones you do not like, perhaps because you dislike the smell or how they make you feel. If you are sensitive or just trying them out for the first time try diluting the essential oil with a carrier oil, such as organic, raw coconut oil. Some people, however, use them without diluting them and have no issue.

Midwives and doulas have come to incorporate essential oils with their work. They are great, all-natural and can be used while pregnant. There are oils that should be used with caution and not at all during pregnancy. (See the list of those not recommended in pregnancy.) However, those you can use produce fantastic results. There are even oils to use postpartum that can help increase breast milk supply, such as fennel and geranium.

In the book *Aromatherapy: Essential Oils in Practice*, Jane Buckle, PHD, RN says, "There are no records of abnormal fetuses or aborted fetuses due to the normal use of essential oils either by topical application or inhalation. There are no records of a few drops of essential oils taken by mouth causing any problem either."[42]

Essential Oils to *Avoid* During Pregnancy

Basil
Birch
Calamus
Cassia
Cinnamon Bark
Hyssop
Idaho Tansy
Jasmine (can start contractions)
Lavendin
Oregano
Rosemary
Sage
Tarragon
Di-Gize
Dragon Time
Exodus II
Grounding
Mister

Essential Oils to Use with *Caution* During Pregnancy

Some women are able to use these oils while others are not.
Heavily dilute them and see how your body reacts.

Angelica
Cedarwood
Chamomile(German/blue)
Cistus
Citronella
Clary Sage (can start labor)
Clove Bud
Cumin (black)
Cypress
Davana
Fennel
Laurel
Marjoram
Mountain Savory
Myrrh
Nutmeg
Rose
Spearmint
Vetiver
Yarrow
Aroma Siez
Clarity
Harmony
ImmuPower
Relieve It
Thieves

I began using essential oils during my third pregnancy and I wish I had used them sooner. In this chapter, when referring to the oils I am only referring to Young Living Essential Oils.

Essential Oil Go To Guide For Birth

HALT EARLY LABOR
LAVENDER-APPLY A FEW DROPS ON THE TUMMY
PEACE AND CALMING-APPLY A FEW DROPS ON THE CHEST
OR DIFFUSE

CALM A LABORING MOM
LAVENDER-RELAXATION, EASE MUSCLE TENSION-
TOPICAL OR DIFFUSE
FRANKINSCENCE-CALM EMOTIONS-TOPICAL OR DIFFUSE
YLANG YLANG-INCREASE CALMNESS, SLOWS BREATHING-
TOPICAL OR DIFFUSE
PEACE AND CALMING-RELAXATION-TOPICAL OR DIFFUSE
BERGAMOT-APPLY TO FOREHEAD AND TEMPLES OR DIFFUSE
GENTLE BABY-CALMS MOM AND BABY, DIFFUSE OR TOPICAL
JOY-LIFT YOUR MOOD BY DIFFUSING OR A DROP ON YOUR
HEART
ORANGE-CAN LIFT YOUR MOOD BY DIFFUSING OR TOPICAL
STRESSAWAY-TAKES THE STRESS AWAY AND CALMS BY
DIFFUSING OR TOPICAL

TO ENCOURAGE LABOR
CLARY SAGE-CAN USE AROMATICALLY, OR ON PRESSURE
POINTS BETWEEN THUMB AND FINGER, TOPS OF
SHOULDERS, INNER ANKLES. WITH CAUTION, SOME
INJEST IN CAPSULE
JASMINE- DIFFUSE OR BOTTOMS OF FEET AND TUMMY
FENNEL-APPLY ON PINKY TOES TO KEEP LABOR GOING
MYRRH-DIFFUSE OR TOPICAL TO PERINEUM DURING
LABOR TO SOFTEN

BREECH OR POSTERIOR POSITION
PEPPERMINT-FOR BREECH-APPLY WITH A CARRIER OIL
AND APPLY AROUND THE TOP CURVE OF THE BELLY

FOR POSTERIOR-APPLY WITH A CARRIER OIL TO THE LOWER BACK

DISCOMFORT
PANAWAY- TOPICALLY TO TUMMY, LOWER BACK OR WHEREVER NEEDED
DEEP RELIEF-TOPICALLY TO TUMMY, LOWER BACK OR WHEREVER NEEDED
VALOR-TOPICALLY ALONG SPINE, HIPS AND ALONG JAWLINE-AN OPEN RELAXED JAW MAKES WAY FOR AN OPEN BIRTH PATH
FRANKINSCENCE-TOPICALLY TO TUMMY OR LOWER BACK
PEPPERMINT-TOPICALLY FOR BACK LABOR

NAUSEA
PEPPERMINT-DIFFUSE OR TOPICALLY OR INGEST
LEMON-IN WATER OR DIFFUSE
ORANGE- IN WATER OR DIFFUSE
DIGIZE-ON STOMACHE OR DIFFUSE
GINGER-DIFFUSE OR ON STOMACHE

STAMINA & ENERGY
VALOR-AROMATIC OR TOPICAL
PEPPERMINT-AROMATIC (MAY SLOW MILK PRODUCTION)
EN-R-GEE-AROMATIC OR TOPICAL
ORANGE-DIFFUSE OR IN WATER TOPICAL
BERGAMOT-DIFFUSE OR TOPICAL
LEMON-DIFFUSE OR IN WATER

PERINEUM CARE
FRANKINSCENCE-TOPICAL- PRIOR TO DELIVERY CAN BE USED DURING PERINEAL MASSAGE- DURING AND AFTER DELIVERY FOR DISCOMFORT/TEARS
HELICHRYSIUM-TOPICAL WITH CARRIER OIL-DURING DELIVERY TO INCREASE ELASTICITY, REDUCE SWELLING

LAVENDER-MIX WITH WATER IN BOTTLE TO USE AFTER GOING TO THE BATHROOM-VERY SOOTHING
GERANIUM-2 DROPS IN WATER, 5 DROPS LAVENDER, WET WASHCLOTH, STORE IN THE FREEZER AND APPY TO SORE AREA

TONE UTERUS
GERANIUM-TOPICALLY
LAVENDER-TOPICALLY
JASMINE-TOPICALLY
YLANG YLANG-TOPICALLY
FRANKINSCENCE-TOPICALLY

INCREASE MILK PRODUCTION
***FENNEL**-APPLY AROUND BREASTS OR 2 DROPS IN A TEASPOON OF HONEY EVERY 2 HOURS, FOLLOW WITH A GLASS OF WATER*
***GERANIUM**-APPLY AROUND BREASTS*

FOR CLEARING THE AIR
***THEIVES**-DIFFUSE*
***PURIFICATION**-DIFFUSE*

POSTPARTUM
DRAGON TIME- BALANCE EMOTIONS AND MOOD SWINGS, CRAMP RELIEF
JOY-HORMONE BALANCE AND STRESS RELIEF
CLARY SAGE-MAY HELP WITH POSTPARTUM BLEEDING AND MOOD
GENTLE BABY- CALMING, IMPROVE APPREARANCE OF SKIN ON TUMMY
PEPPERMINT-PUT A DROP IN THE TOILET, HELPS WITH URINATION

FOR HEMMORAGING/EXESSIVE BLEEDING- IF A HISTORY OF BLEEDING THEY CAN BE USED A WEEK PRIOR TO BIRTH. IF MEDICAL CARE IS NOT AVAILABLE...THEY ARE GOOD TO KNOW IN A DESPARATE SITUATION
*FRANINSCENCE-*APPLY TO BIG TOES ON THE OUTER SIDE
GENTLE BABY- APPLY ON LOWER BACK, BELLY AND INSIDE OF ANKLES
HELYCHRYSIUM- APPLY ON LOWER BACK, BELLY AND INSIDE OF ANKLES

There are some oils which may prep your body and support your reproductive system before conception. Geranium and Calendula can help support and balance hormones, regulating your cycle. Clary Sage can be good for both men and women by boosting libido and hormone support when trying to conceive. Ginger is good for circulatory system support. Basil is also another oil which may boost libido or go with your favorite scent. My husband likes Abundance as cologne!

Popular Young Living Essential Oils and Uses

One of the most versatile oils many use daily is Peppermint oil. During pregnancy Peppermint oil can be used for most any need that occurs as the body changes like supporting the muscular and skeletal systems as the body changes and discomfort arises. It supports the digestive system for occasional constipation or tummy issues. Respiratory and nervous system can also be supported with peppermint during pregnancy. Feeling overheated, it can cool you down and be an energy booster. It is great when used during the first trimester. I put a drop on a damp washcloth, or put a drop in my water or tea. Some women also like to use the Lemon essential oil the same way, add a drop or two to water. Citrus oils of any type—Lime, Orange, Tangerine, and Lemon—are popular to support the digestive system. (Citrus oils can cause sun sensitivity so use caution) Some midwives have even had success at making sure the baby is in proper head down position by using Peppermint oil. If we all tried that and had successful outcomes, think about how many C-sections could be prevented! As soon as you are four weeks away from your due date, you may want to stop using Peppermint oil, because it can halt breast milk production in some women.

Clary Sage can support women during PMS and contains natural phytoestrogens. Some take it only before conception, but consult your doctor on this particular oil. Clary Sage also helps induce labor and is to be used with caution.

Another oil that I used during pregnancy for stress related discomforts, tension and jaw issues is Valor. When the jaw is relaxed so will the body and be relaxed to birth. Some women also use it during labor in the transition phase. It is very versatile—it can help ground you and alleviate hip and back discomfort when applied to sacrum and hips. For these reasons, it is very popular and you will want to have it on hand. I, for instance, used it daily during my third trimester as my back and hips started to shift from the weight of the baby. I relied on Valor alongside my chiropractic treatments with great results.

Some women experience swelling during pregnancy. This is especially brutal when it is hot in the summer. You can put Lavender, or Geranium in coconut oil and massage into swollen ankles or puffy fingers for relief.

If you have a love affair with sugar, try Ocotea oil. Many people use it to help maintain normal blood sugar levels…including me. You can take Ocotea in a capsule or put 5 drops in a teaspoon of coconut oil and take it once or twice a day. If I ate more carbs one day, for instance, I would take two spoonfuls. Apple cider vinegar also lowers blood sugar levels.

Let us talk about stretch marks, ladies. Some of us never get them while others do. People have had good outcomes at avoiding them by using Frankincense, Myrrh, Lavender, and Gentle Baby. Gentle Baby also reduces stress and helps you bond with the baby. You could diffuse it after delivery or during. Some even use it on a baby's bottom.

A great tip is to add an essential oil to your olive oil when you do the Perineal Massage, I recommend Frankincense. It can help with elasticity of the skin.[43] Also, can be used to anoint the baby.

If you think you are having symptoms of early labor, try putting a few drops of Peace and Calming on your chest and Lavender on your stomach. As always, contact the midwife or ob-gyn if you are having true symptoms of early labor. Peace and Calming is great to use throughout pregnancy to calm and de-stress you, as well. The scent is mild and a lot of women like it as a perfume! It helps to calm babies too! Lavender is also good for this as well.

To clear the air while at the hospital some women diffuse Purification. You can also take Thieves now that you have had the baby. Thieves is not always recommended during pregnancy but may be tolerated for some women. It contains Cinnamon Bark oil which is to be avoided during pregnancy and may even cause premature labor.[44]

During labor, Pan Away is a great oil to use to deal with any discomfort you may be having, but it is not to be used during pregnancy.

Fennel is used to support lactation in place of nursing tea. You may not need any extra help for milk to come in after a couple days after birth but it is good to know it is there!

If you develop breast issues—or feel engorged when your milk comes in, some women have success with one drop of Geranium. I suggest you mix one drop of Lavender with a pint and a half of water, then dip a cloth in the liquid to make a cold compress and apply to the breasts.

There is a great book called *Gentle Babies* by Debra Raybern, which includes a lot of information on using Young Living Oils for pregnancy, childbirth, and young children. I relied on this book to help incorporate oil use throughout my pregnancy and even into labor. During pregnancy I found it useful to put Peppermint on my shoulders or wherever I felt my body needed support from pregnancy related discomfort. Lemon oil in water or peppermint added for a refreshing drink. I might add that I feel the Peppermint helped me avoid having to sleep propped up on a pillow like I had during my last pregnancies due to the baby pushing on my tummy. I used Valor on my jaw to relax and on my back. Peace and Calming and Stress Away did the trick to remove any feelings of worry or stress!

Lavender and Frankincense became my favorite to put on my face. I applied these before bed and woke with a smoother face. Some nights I mixed the oils with coconut oil and applied it topically to my face to counteract dryness.

As I approached my due date, occasionally before bed I used Gentle Baby on my tummy or Lavender.

My Story: How I Used Essential Oils Leading up to, During, and After Labor

When my due date came and went with my third pregnancy and my doctor mentioned the term "induction," I began to research what I could do to induce naturally. During my second pregnancy, I had gestational diabetes. I induced with eggplant Parmesan, Evening Primrose oil, sex, walking, and acupuncture. By doing those things, I went into labor on my due date with my second child.

With this last pregnancy, my third, I had a lot of work that I needed to complete. The main goal was finishing this book! Instead of inducing, I decided to let nature take its course—that is until I reached 41 weeks. Then I decided to use Young Living Essential Oils in addition to the other methods that I had been successful with in the past. On Saturday, when I suspected that labor was approaching—I had a mild backache—a friend, Pam, brought me Young Living Clary Sage oil. From what I researched, it said to use it with caution, because it could have different effects on different people.

I took a few whiffs of Young Living Clary Sage oil in the afternoon and evening. I also consumed an eggplant parmesan dish with lots of herbs and spices and took Evening Primrose oil. When I woke up Sunday morning and nothing had happened, I applied Clary Sage to three pressure points known in Chinese Medicine to induce labor: points on my hand, leg, and shoulders.

That day, my daughter and I went for a swim! Before I left the house, I applied more Clary Sage oil on the pressure points and Peace and Calming on my chest and neck to relax. I mostly floated around the pool and walked back and forth in the pool. Still, nothing! For lunch, I ate foods I knew could induce labor: eggplant parmesan and pineapple with the core. Around 2:30 pm, I felt a little twinge in my back. A few intermittent back twinges later, I thought I might be going into labor, even though it didn't feel like my previous labors. Instead, these contractions were very mild and erratic. It mostly felt like the baby was moving about stretching.

I called my Doula and began timing contractions. When I noticed each contraction was about six minutes to seven minutes apart, I got excited. My family left the pool and ate dinner, and I had my husband pack his bag while I took a quick shower. My Doula, Kathy, arrived at about 6:00 pm and, shortly after, I requested she insert a few acupuncture needles to calm me. I still was not in intense labor or feeling pain during contractions. On a scale of 1-10 they were maybe a 5 or 6. During this wait-time I kept applying Peace and Calming to relax. After my Doula was with me for a bit, I began using Pan Away. Pan Away is used when you are in real labor.

For this third pregnancy, my husband and I choose a different hospital, Stony Brook University Hospital, was a better choice than the hospital I used last time because, it has a reputation for being very supportive for all natural, drug-free births. Although my last birth was all-natural and drug free, the nursing staff was not very supportive. This lack of support sparked me to change hospitals and see a midwife instead of an ob-gyn, too. However, by choosing this hospital, we had an hour-long drive from our house. With my Doula following closely behind us, we drove. I filled the car with the smell of Stress Away, Peace and Calming, Pan Away, and Valor. Fifteen minutes after we left home, we all piled into the same car. My Doula immediately deduced that I was transitioning quickly and my contractions were much closer together. Between contractions she and I applied oils!

As we approached the hospital, I felt the need to do the deep 'aww' sound that numbed my tummy during the last birth. No one knew I was a little worried that I might have this baby in the car. I was more nervous because I was not wearing my seat belt, but rather leaning backwards over the back seat. At two miles away it felt like I might have to push! During one contraction it actually felt like the baby was pushing and that my body wanted to push with him!

The oils I applied were especially helpful in calming me and helping me maintain a level head. For instance, when we finally got to the hospital, my mood was mild, and my mind clear enough to know I did not want a wheelchair. I remembered that sitting does not help—gravity helps the baby descend. I also declined the hospital gown and opted for my lucky bra. Finally, I firmly decided to lean on the bed, still standing, with my chest and arms stretched out. This was the most comfortable position for me during my last birth and for this one as well. All this time, my husband set up music, my diffuser and spread Peace and Calming throughout my hospital room. This helped me feel ready to give birth.

When the doctor checked me while I was on all fours, she said I was almost fully dilated at nine and a half centimeters. I was shocked by how quickly I got to delivery and how minimized my pain felt. I attribute this partly to the Peace and Calming, Valor, Pan Away, and Stress Away I kept applying during the car ride between contractions. I also know the acupuncture needles, seven weeks of listening to Marie Mongan Hypnobirthing CDs, and the support of my Doula helped me transition quickly and calmly.

Upon a very intense contraction, I got off my hands and knees, stood up and began to lean on the bed, waiting for more contractions and my cue to push. With a few more contractions and pushing, my baby boy arrived at exactly 9:00 pm on August 17th, 2014. We delayed the clamping until the cord stopped pulsing blood into his little body. He began breastfeeding soon after. I was so elated with my second all natural, drug-free vaginal birth! I had no tearing, no need for ice, and was pretty comfortable once I decided to sit on the bed! We diffused Gentle Baby oil in our private room and alternated that with Peace and Calming to have a peaceful experience, bonding with the baby.

Though this hospital's protocol after birth is to give a woman Pitocin—a standard drug given at most hospitals to stop bleeding and "help" the uterus contract—I declined. Pitocin is known to result in stronger uterine contractions after labor. Instead, breastfeeding and massaging the uterus are natural ways to induce uterine contractions and cease bleeding. But once I began to bleed more than the nurses and doctors liked, they began to push the Pitocin. Luckily, my doula consulted my *Gentle Babies* book and applied Frankincense to the tips of my big toes. Wouldn't you know it, Frankincense oil in combination with massaging my uterus and breastfeeding got the bleeding to stop! I had my perfect birth. I might have used Pitocin should my other methods have failed, and I advise you to take the advice of the experts around you. But, for me, these methods luckily worked, naturally as God intended!

For those first time moms out there, when you do have your second and third baby, be warned the uterus contracting is more painful after you give birth. It feels like a really painful menstrual cramp. Some women can tolerate this step of healing drug-free, while others opt for Tylenol, Advil, or Motrin. While many suggest breastfeeding women should not take medication, if pain inhibits your ability to care for your baby, a couple doses may be worth a try. After 12-24 hours the cramping stops, and you will hopefully not need anything additional for pain. I did try applying Pan Away for a while on my lower abdomen, but stopped when I got worried it might irritate the baby when he rested on my chest.

I really enjoyed using the Young Living oils throughout pregnancy and birth, and continue to use them for my family. This is my story and how I used the oils in 2014. You should use oils as directed on the label or research more online. They have really become a part of our everyday life. Having such a holistic lifestyle, they were the missing link that I found to use for just about everything you can imagine! You can contact me if you would like to learn more on Young Living Oils for you, your family and pets as well!

CHAPTER TWELVE: WALDORF PHILOSOPHY AND NON-TOXIC NATURAL BABY PRODUCTS

What is the Waldorf Philosophy? Rudolph Steiner started this philosophy of teaching in 1919. To Steiner, the human being is threefold with body, spirit, and soul. Children also have three different stages of development: From birth to 7-years-old (early childhood), 7- to 14-years-old (middle childhood), and 14- to 18-years-old (adolescence). To him, children should be supported through age-appropriate content during each stage. The Waldorf Philosophy, then, seeks to understand and support each childhood stage fully to help each child develop in a healthy way.

We stumbled upon a local Waldorf school when my daughter was 20 months old and found it complimented our parenting style perfectly. Less is more, in a way. What a joy it was to learn that the Waldorf natural way of learning includes having natural, non-toxic toys and baby products on hand for little ones. The classroom, for example, was filled with wood toys and cotton or wool dolls. The children learn by doing. We fell in love. It was a nontoxic environment that served organic food and used non-toxic cleaning products. What a perfect match for our child. As I've mentioned before, we never wanted enormous amounts of plastic toys in our home or an overabundance of "stuff" that gets thrown in landfills. It turns out that our way or doing things coincided with what they are teaching in their parent-child classes, which continue on to nursery school, kindergarten, and beyond. There are Waldorf Schools all over the world.

"Throughout, the approach stresses the role of the imagination in learning and places a strong value on integrating intellectual, practical, and artistic themes.

The educational philosophy's overarching goal is to develop free[45], morally[46] responsible, and integrated individuals equipped with a high degree of social competence."

The older child learns all sorts of crafts and activities—that are not usually offered in school today—such as knitting, woodworking, and quilting. They begin to learn a second language in kindergarten, such as French or German. Music and art are big parts of the Waldorf education, because they also encourage children to use their imaginations. Subjects are not taught, read about, or tested: they are experienced. The child is also not "graded," but rather their progress is discussed at parent-teacher conferences.

Waldorf schools can be the perfect environment for your child. They are growing more and more popular as parents seek an alternative education that inspires creativity and imagination with age-appropriate content for the learning process.

There are also Waldorf Homeschooling programs you can purchase online if homeschooling is a fit for your family. These include:

www.christoperushomeschool.com
www.waldorfessentials.com
www.live-education.com

While there are many books written on parenthood, not all will follow a simple, natural, philosophy. Some books that you will find helpful on your journey to parenthood are:

Beyond the Rainbow Bridge
You Are Your Childs First Teacher
Simplicity Parenting
The Attachment Parenting Handbook, Dr. Sears
Heaven on Earth: A Handbook for Parents of Young Children

Non-toxic Baby Items

During first pregnancies some women can get a little nutty about what they buy. I know I did. Researching all of the non-toxic items and having as many organic items of clothing, burp clothes, bibs, towels, bedding, and so forth became my mission. This was back in the summer of 2009 when organic baby items were just emerging. Searching stores high and low, I found all sorts of organic items. I knew these items would reduce the amount of the toxins I was exposed to during the remainder of my pregnancy, and be safe for my new baby.

Today, due to demand, there are many more organic options, as clothing suppliers now make clothes that fit children past their first year of life. Cotton and wool are the best options for babies and children. Polyester should be avoided, as should anything synthetic. There are many more places where you can find organic bedding, towels, burp clothes, and bibs, too.

We all must acknowledge that other people will purchase new items for your baby. With this in mind, well before you register for baby things, let family members know if you will be adopting the "less is more" lifestyle and include organic and non-toxic items to your registry. This is the greenest way to be!

The marketing of toys and gadgets for babies and kids is overwhelming and makes us think we need everything we see. Many of the "things" over-stimulate, and are really just more for the parent. Truth be told, the majority of the products are not tested properly for safety and are often recalled. Believe it or not, many baby and toddler items contain toxic flame-retardants and other hazardous chemicals. Neither the toy companies nor the government regulate chemicals allowed in products, so you never know what you are buying unless you do your research. We, the consumer who only wants the best for our baby or others' babies, must keep this in mind.

We want our babies to play with toys that they can put in their mouths without fearing they might ingest something toxic. This is why it is best to choose toys made from organic cloth, wool, or natural, unpainted wood.

It is also better for the environment if you steer clear of plastic toys and gadgets. How long do you actually use these toys? They eventually break and end up in a landfill polluting the earth. Embracing "less is more" goes along with a Waldorf approach to parenting, which many parents turn to as they see the effects of "too much too soon."

Favorite Non-Toxic Baby Items

Young America Furniture-non-toxic cribs, dressers, beds,

Naturepedic latex mattress, changing pad, bassinet pad

Organic or Oeko-tek certified sheets for the crib (Pottery Barn Kids, Land of Nod)

Glass bottles (Lifefactory)

Stainless bowls (Green Sprouts, Think baby)

Organic or Oeko-tek onesies, pjs, and clothes (Hanna Anderson, Under the Nile, Katie Quinn, Gerber Organic. Various stores have organic lines, just ask or look online.)

Orbit car seats (pricey but non-toxic)

UPPAbaby stroller with non-toxic fabric (use the bassinet feature as much as possible to allow baby to move freely)

Bugaboo stroller with wheel a board for toddler (use bassinet feature as well)

Stokke highchair (wood and can be used as child beyond toddlerhood)

Ergo Baby Organic Carrier (note, do not use for extended time, babies need to move freely)

Organic bibs, burp clothes and towels, blankets (Swaddle designs, Burt's Bees, Under the Nile)

Green Sprouts by Iplay bath mat (PVC free), food storage, organic burp clothes, teethers, rattles.

Honest Diapers and wipes

Nature Baby Care training pants and toddler wipes

Earth Mama Angel baby shampoo, body wash, nipple cream

Badger Sunscreen

Boiron colic drops, teething drops

Young Living Essential Oils (Gentle Baby, Peace and Calming, Lavender, KidScents oil collection)

Wood toys, teethers (Nova Natural, Plan Toys)

Organic, cloth toys (miYim, Dandelion, Green Sprouts)

Amber necklace for teething (Nova Naturals, Amazon)

Organic nursing cover and pillow

Under3essentials.com

Novanatural.com

Palumba.com

Magiccabin.com

Giggle.com

By staying green and minimizing the amount of stuff in your home, you will do your baby and the planet a huge favor. Choose high-quality items that are nontoxic, won't break before your first child is done playing with them, and can be used over and over, generation after generation. Think before you buy: Does my baby really need this?

CHAPTER THIRTEEN: RESTORE YOUR BODY DURING THE FOURTH TRIMESTER AND BEYOND

What is the fourth trimester? According to Dr. Harvey Karp, the fourth trimester is the three months after the baby is born. You can never cuddle too much or feed too much during this time. Feeding on demand can be normal for babies since they need their nutrients. Co-sleeping may be just what your baby needs to keep from crying and being colicky. This fourth trimester is an adjustment for you and your baby. Now you need to restore your health and heal by eating properly, because you are still eating for two.

Although indulging in foods you missed when you were pregnant might tempt you, try not to give in. Try to continue with the healthy eating habits that you have created. Maybe give yourself one reward that you have been missing for nine months, but do not get in the habit of indulging in unhealthy foods on a regular basis. You will definitely feel worse physically, if you start to eat processed foods again. Stay strong—now is a time to recharge and replenish your body so you can heal and make healthy milk for your baby.

What to Eat to Restore Your Body

Healthy, organic food is just as important postpartum as it was during pre-conception and pregnancy. Your body has lost a lot of blood and is trying to balance your hormones. First off, you want to eat foods that are rich in iron. These include: Liver, Red Meat (such as

Bison, Venison or Beef), Caviar, Egg Yolks, Sesame Butter/Tahini, (healthy sustainably raised) Clams/Oysters/Mussels, Sardines, Cacao Powder, Sundried Tomatoes, Sunflower Seeds, Pumpkin Seeds, Thyme, Parsley, Spinach, Swiss Chard, Beans (such as Lentils, Chickpeas, Kidney, Pinto, Butter, Peas, or Haricot), Curry Powder, Nuts (such as Almonds, Cashews, Brazil Nuts, Walnuts), Sulfite-free Dried Apricots, and Quinoa.

You also do not want to drink tea with your meal as it can inhibit the absorption of iron. Because you've lost a lot of iron with the loss of blood during delivery, it is important to give your body its best chance to replenish and absorb iron. For this reason, if you are drinking a lactating tea, drink it between meals.

What To Eat to Produce Breast Milk and Other Breastfeeding Tips

Breastfeeding is by far the greenest option for feeding your newborn. You do not have to keep up with the demands of buying formula and you can also go without bottles for as long as you wish. No clean up! There is a great sense of accomplishment that comes with this, too. Breast milk has the best nutrients and antibodies to fight off viruses for your baby, and it is free.

Foods to Promote Breast milk Production

Oatmeal
Spinach
Carrots
Hummus
Non-GMO Papaya
Asparagus
Green Beans
Yams
Sweet Potatoes
Dandelion Greens and Leafy Green Vegetables

Peas
Apricots
Wild Sustainable Salmon
Water
Parsley
Fennel and Fenugreek
Sesame Seeds
Raw Almonds
Cashews
Macadamia Nuts
Avocados
Coconut Water
Lactation Tea Blends-Mountain Rose Herbs Nurse-Me Rhyme
Barley Water
Garlic
Onion
Ginger
Marjoram
Basil
Anise
Dill
Caraway
Turmeric
Spirulina
Brewer's Yeast

Note: If any of these foods don't agree with you, they may not agree with your baby.

To help with milk production, you can drink Traditional Medicinals Mother's Milk tea. You can bring it to the hospital and drink a few cups a day. Then, drink it every other day if needed. It works great and tastes good, especially if you add Stevia to sweeten it. Mountain Rose Herbs Nursing Tea called Nurse-Me Rhyme Tea is also a great loose-leaf, organic option.

What to avoid eating in order to prevent colic and fussiness seems to vary amongst babies. One thing a majority of women have in common, though, is that they must stop eating dairy because it negatively affects the infant. Some babies do not like it when their moms eat beans, broccoli, or cauliflower. Others do not do well when a mom has caffeine, which new mothers should avoid anyway. Avoid peppermint and parsley because it can halt milk production. This is not true for all women, though.

Remember to avoid alcohol or use the test strips to check your milk for alcohol after you have a drink. Wait time differs for each person, because we each have a different metabolism when it comes to alcohol. Testing is crucial: We don't want the baby to get any alcohol into his system. Each baby is different and you just have to see what foods work for you. If you have a family history of certain food allergies, your baby may be allergic as well. Common allergens are things such as wheat, eggs, corn, dairy, shellfish, peanuts, and soy.

If you plan on breastfeeding, there are certain things that make life easier. First you need Earth Mama Angel Baby Nipple Cream. There are other brands, but I especially like this one because it is lanolin free, organic, and the breast doesn't need to be washed off before feeding your baby. Putting a little of your own milk on the nipple works well, too. You can also use raw coconut oil to moisturize. If you get a breast infection (mastitis) or if milk comes in and your breasts become engorged, you can use on drop of Geranium oil (Young Living Brand) and one drop of Lavender (Young Living Brand). Combine these drops with a pint and a half of cool water, soak a washcloth in the mixture, and use it as a cold compress. Women have also used cold cabbage leaves applied to the breast!

A breast pump is great to have. They are pricey, but well worth it, especially if you will be going back to work and need to pump. I used a popular brand pump, which is great for pumping and also comes in handy if you want to mix milk with baby cereal once your baby can eat solid foods. Though you can express milk by hand, it is not easy. A pump of some sort is good to have. Brands which are better than the one I had and have a closed system which I am told is better, are Spectra 2,

Hygeia Enjoi, Bailey Nurture III and Ameda Purely Yours. Check with your insurance because some now pay for breast pumps.

As far as bottles, the BPA-free bottles that come with the breast pump are what a lot of women use. You may want to use glass instead of plastic in light of the recent backlash on BPA-free bottles, which suggests that some still contain harmful chemicals. For working moms who need to store and freeze milk, use plastic for storage only, since heating plastic might be hazardous. Heating the plastic bottle with milk in it, for instance, can often be an issue. If this is the case, you can always store milk in plastic, then reheat it in glass after it thaws and serve it in glass. Consult a lactation specialist on bottles because research is emerging everyday on safety.

Nursing bras and tanks are great to have in your wardrobe. You will want to have one per day or you will smell like sour milk. Nursing tanks for the winter are good to keep you extra warm. Instead of using disposable breast pads, which fill up landfills, opt for organic, cotton, reusable breast pads. When nursing in public, a button down shirt can work great. For nursing tops, I recommend cotton, wool, or hemp if you have a fussy baby for easy access! These fabrics are best if they are not washed with any harmful detergents. Remember, your baby is inhaling whatever is on your body or clothes.

A good nursing pillow is helpful when you are nursing at home. Be warned, though, popular brands tend to be made from toxic materials, such as polyurethane foam! Look for an organic pillow made with natural fillers. You can also use a latex pillow, or lay down to nurse, which I find so relaxing. Remember, women have breastfed for ages without a nursing pillow.

Whatever option is best for you, please give breastfeeding a try! For help, you can contact your local Le Leche League if your hospital does not have a lactation consultant. The first few days or weeks can be a challenge, but once you learn the ins and outs of breastfeeding it becomes rewarding. In the long-run you are doing what is best for your baby and providing milk in the greenest possible way.

If there is some reason you cannot breastfeed—some women can't breastfeed because they take necessary medications or for other reasons—don't fret. There are options for bottle-feeding that do not include over the counter formula (these contain GMOs and other mysterious ingredients). There are a few on the market that are suitable. Organic is best. If you like you can make your own super easy and healthy formula. In fact, many moms are now making their own formula when they can no longer breastfeed or are trying to wean their baby. Below, you'll find a great recipe for Goat Milk Formula. There are also many other homemade formula recipes you can find online. This one happens to be what my child thrived on as a supplement upon weaning. I found it from Mt. Capra.

GOAT MILK FORMULA

1 Tablespoon Powdered Goat Milk
1 teaspoon Organic Raw Coconut Oil
1 teaspoon Organic Cold Pressed Olive Oil
1/8 teaspoon Organic Molasses (iron)
Liquid multivitamin dosage as directed (with folate, not folic acid)
4 ounces hot water/4 ounces cool water
1/4 teaspoon Probiotic Powder for Infants (Klaire Labs)

This is just one option. Remember, infants have different requirements than adults or young children. Do your research and see what is best for your baby. Consult a naturopath or nutritionist who is familiar with homemade formulas and the nutrients your baby needs. The ingredients you are using will be much healthier than the majority of the formulas on the market and, most likely, less expensive.

Now that you have an idea of what to eat to recharge your body, you can plan ahead before your baby arrives. Planning to breastfeed is the greenest option. Having a few necessary nursing items will make breastfeeding easier as well.

Maintaining Your Green Lifestyle for You, the Earth, and Your Future Children

Along with eating healthy after pregnancy you also need to care for yourself emotionally and physically. The day you have dreamed about is here, and you have your healthy baby! Focus on the baby and bonding time. Do not, however, forget to focus on your health. The amount of energy and work your body has gone through in the past nine to ten months has been tremendous. You should give yourself a big pat on the back for a job well done. Now is a time to rest and recuperate as well as care for your little bundle of joy.

Enlist the help of family and friends to do some cooking and cleaning in the first few weeks. Some people even hire postpartum doulas to help during this transitional time. These weeks tend to be the most draining on parents with a lot of sleep deprivation—having a baby is a big change. Before baby comes, freeze meals ahead of time for a quick-fix meal you can eat after you give birth. Take-out is not the best option, unless you know the food is GMO-free and, hopefully, organic. Your body needs the best nutrients to heal and to breastfeed.

In addition, if you plan on having more children, staying on a healthy-eating routine will enable your body to heal and replenish itself for another pregnancy. Maintaining a healthy lifestyle can make a second conception much easier. One thing to keep in mind as you bond with baby: Less is more. Too many visitors and the baby may become over-stimulated and be unable to get optimal rest. This means mom can't achieve optimal rest, either.

Wanting to return to your pre-pregnancy weight? Be patient, your body will return soon. This is something some women worry about after pregnancy. My best advice is, DO NOT WORRY about it. Enjoy your baby! Eventually the baby weight will come off.

All of your skin changes and discolorations will go back to normal during this time, too. Stretch marks may take a little longer. You will also bleed for up to six weeks postpartum. Your breasts may become engorged if you are breastfeeding, but they soon will go down as feeding becomes regular. The cramping you feel after delivery is your uterus shrinking back down to its pre-pregnancy size. These things are all normal. You may be constipated after delivery if you have had an epidural. In addition, your hair may thin a little due to hormone fluctuations. These hormones may even cause you to breakout a little temporarily. You might also wake up in a sweat. All of these things are to be expected and will be temporary. If you are having trouble not leaking when you sneeze or laugh, something that also happens during pregnancy, remember to continue to do Kegel exercises for a few weeks or months to strengthen muscles that control your bladder. You will be your old self again! It took 40 weeks to grow the baby, give your body a chance and it will heal.

Lack of sleep is something your body has a hard time adjusting to. Sleep when baby sleeps and put off doing housework or checking emails during this time so you can rest. Too little sleep can also affect your immune system.

Remember to wear comfortable clothes and give yourself three to six months to fully recharge. Becoming a parent can be harder for some people and easier for others. Everyone adjusts at a different pace, so you should not stress if it takes you a little longer. Having the first baby is the hardest, because you need to adjust to sleep changes and lifestyle changes. With each child the adjustments get much easier for anyone wanting a big family!

If these physical changes are getting you down, look at your baby to remember it was all worth it! If you feel sadder than normal, you might have post-partum depression (PPD). If you think you might be suffering from PPD, seek professional advice. It can also be helpful to join a support group for new moms who are breastfeeding or living a holistic lifestyle. One group that I really enjoy is the Holistic Moms Network. You can find moms like you who attend the monthly meetings. You can also listen to speakers and discuss topics that are relevant to your parenting choices. Look them up at www.holisticmoms.org.

Your Next Baby

Now that you have had your first child you may think that if you can have one, it should be easy to have a second. This is not always the case. Many women who breastfeed do not ovulate until they have weaned the baby. Remember, though, there is still a chance you could become pregnant even if you breastfeed. For those moms who have "Irish twins" or even babies spaced very close together, this is a big challenge and exhausting. Your body needs time to heal after birth so use caution if you want to prevent pregnancy. Also, you want to bond with the new baby for at least a year to savor every quiet moment.

When it is time for you to try to conceive a second child, you should eat green and organic foods. If you stay on this path—and don't fall back into old habits after your first child—you will have a much easier time. Some women, for instance, struggle for months or years trying to conceive a second or third child because they fall into the rut of eating take-out or processed foods, do not get enough sleep, or are just run down after their first baby arrives. Taking care of yourself so you can take care of your family is key! Try rereading this book after you have your first child to remind yourself of all the healthy things you need to be doing in order to promote healthy eggs and sperm for your next pregnancy.

By taking the extra time to eat healthy meals for you and your first child, you are doing your family an enormous favor. Children mimic what they see. If you pull through the drive through, they will want fast food. But by showing your children how to eat healthy, nutritious, low-sugar meals, you are building up their healthy immune systems and teaching them good habits.

Children will even eat salad! Surprised? Eating healthy also means fewer trips to the doctor and, hopefully, an easier second conception for you and your husband! Going Green is a huge step for some. Just know that implementing even small changes will help your health, your family, the planet, and future generations!

Good luck on your journey of *Going Green Before You Conceive!*

CHAPTER FOURTEEN: THE GOING GREEN FOOD PLAN

When deciding what to eat for fertility, you will need to take into consideration your own personal health and preferences. Are you trying to conceive a boy or girl? That will determine if your diet should be acidic or alkaline. Are you suffering from PCOS or endometriosis? Then you will need to avoid gluten, dairy, and red meats. If you are diabetic or have a family history of diabetes, you will need to watch your portions of fruit, grains, beans, lentils, and corn in order to control your blood sugar. Do you have a thyroid condition? If so, you should avoid foods that can affect your thyroid, especially raw vegetables such as broccoli, cauliflower, kale, cabbage and Brussels sprouts.

Everyone needs to eat with their own personal health in mind. There is no one size fits all fertility diet plan since each woman and man has their own body chemistry, which can include its own set of health issues that need to be taken into consideration very carefully. There are, however, foods that will boost fertility. You can see if some of them will work for you.

Fertility Favorite Foods

All foods should be Organic/Free Range/ NON- GMO/Non-toxic environments for seafood.

Livers—chicken, beef
Pâté of duck liver, chicken liver
Oysters

Red meat
Lamb
Turkey
Chicken—white and dark meat
Sardines
Eggs—whites and yolk
Almonds, Almond butter
Brazil nuts
Pumpkin seeds
Sesame seeds
Sunflower seeds
Spinach
Kale
Swiss chard
Bok choy
Asparagus
Garlic
Onions
Cauliflower
Celery
Cabbage
Brussels sprouts
Broccoli
Radish
Red peppers
Sweet potatoes
Green peas
Lentils
Mung beans
Pumpkins
Beets
Sauerkraut
Pickles
Coconut oil (raw)
Butter

Ghee
Olive oil (cold-pressed)
Avocado oil
Cinnamon
Water
Red raspberry tea (loose leaf organic)
Decaf green or white tea (loose leaf organic)
Pineapples
Strawberries
Bananas
Citrus fruits—oranges, grapefruits, lemons, limes, tangerines
Kiwi
Blueberries
Tomato

This sample is meant to give you an idea of what foods to eat so you are getting a variety of the nutrients, fats, and minerals needed for conception. If you are beginning to cook from scratch for the first time, it's a good idea to make meals that can be reheated as leftovers for lunch the next day. This way, you only make a meal once but can eat it two or three times. Reheating in the oven is best; never microwave! The process changes the molecules in the food, and research indicates it is not good for the food or your health.[47] Making larger meals in order to have leftovers is especially helpful once baby arrives and time to cook is limited.

During pregnancy, it is important to eat a lot of protein, but be sure to include lots of veggies and a smaller amount of carbs, starches, and fruit to maintain blood sugar levels. When you are eating something with more carbs like pancakes, French toast, or oatmeal, be sure to include protein so that you feel full faster and don't over-indulge.

Sample Diet Ideas

Breakfast

Eggs (hard-boiled, fried, scrambled, egg salad, egg/Manchego/veggie
frittata, omelet)
Chia/Hemp Cereal
Turkey bacon (nitrate free-Applegate farms)
Kale smoothie (see Recipe)
Buckwheat pancakes with turkey bacon (Applegate farms) with honey
Banana/almond pancakes
French toast (gluten-free bread-Rudi's) with turkey bacon (Applegate
farms) with honey
Oatmeal with nuts of your choice, add honey and cinnamon

Lunch and Dinner

Enchiladas with chicken, beef, or beans
Chicken Mexicana
Chicken soup
Chicken livers with apple and sage
Bone broth from beef bones
Almond butter black bean pasta (as a side dish)
Sardine pesto
Gluten-free bison lasagna
Scallops with bok choy, green pea puree
Venison with sweet potato mash and Swiss chard
Roasted onions and garlic go great with any meal!!!
Side dishes of quinoa, beans or lentils are good and last in the refrigerator
for a couple days.

Once a Week:
- Chicken livers (For those who are turning up their nose, your
body will love it for fertility; try my recipe with Fresh Sage)

- Red meat
- Lamb
- Venison
- Low-mercury fish (you can also have these every other week)

Twice a Week:
- Chicken
- Turkey

Once Before Ovulation:
- Raw oysters (these are good for zinc if they are of good quality and ensured to be toxin-free), pumpkin seeds, or sesame seeds for their zinc content. (Not ideal to cook zinc-containing foods.)
- Pineapple with the core at ovulation

Eggs.... as much as you like! Yolks are so healthy as well. The more yellow and orange the yolks are in appearance, the better nutrients. Organic or pasture-raised is best. While the cost is more, you are getting more nutrients. You can also find eggs at farmers markets or a health food store. Quality and color of the yolk is key.

Vegetables of all varieties should be eaten at all meals. Green and leafy is a big plus. Avoid white potatoes, white rice, and limit corn as it can raise blood sugar levels. Try my Kale smoothie recipe to incorporate greens at breakfast or make a spinach omelet or veggie frittata.

Pineapple at the time of ovulation and for about a week after is recommended, since it contains the extract Bromelain, which can help with implantation. Eat small portions of the core, where the highest concentration is, but be careful not to eat excessively as that can cause the opposite effect. One or two fresh pineapple slices per day should contain enough Bromelain. Also Brazil nuts during ovulation for about five days as mentioned earlier in the book.

Favorite Fertility Snacks

Olives

Nuts and Seeds
It's best to find raw nuts, seeds, and butters that have not been roasted. Nuts.com is a great resource, or you can buy (preferably organic) nuts and soak them to make your own nut butter.
    Brazil nuts (selenium)
    Chia seeds, flax seeds, hemp seeds, walnuts (omega-3)
    Pumpkin seeds, sesame seeds, tahini (zinc, iron)
    Almonds, almond butter, sunflower seeds, sun-butter (vitamin E)

Organic Cheese
    Manchego sheep cheese (with gluten-free crackers)
    Goat cheese (with tomatoes)

Pesto with veggies

Fruit with nuts of your choice

Paleo banana bread or pumpkin bread with grass fed butter or almond butter

Favorite Gluten-Free Recipes to Boost Conception and Beyond

Chia cereal
Serves 2

Ingredients:

3 Tbs chia seeds
3 Tbs hemp seeds
1 ripe banana
Almond milk / milk of choice (no soy!)

Directions:

Cover the seeds with milk, and make as creamy and moist as you like. Stir and enjoy. You can also make this the night before, and store for a day for the kids.

Banana Almond Pancakes
Serves 4

Ingredients:

4 ripe bananas
4 organic eggs
1½ cups organic almond meal/flour from nuts.com
½ cup organic coconut flour
1 tsp baking soda
½ tsp salt
2 pats of organic butter for pan
Cinnamon to garnish

Directions:

Mash 4 ripe bananas in a bowl. In a separate bowl, beat 4 eggs. Add the eggs and bananas together. Add the almond meal, coconut flour, baking soda and salt. Stir well. In a pan, melt butter on medium heat. Drop the batter in spoonfuls of 4-5 in a pan. Cook for 3 minutes on each side. Plate and sprinkle with cinnamon if you like. These pancakes are really sweet enough and do not really require honey, maple syrup or agave. You can make extra pancakes and refrigerate to reheat the next day in the pan.

Kale Smoothie Recipe for Boy Conception
Serves 2

Ingredients:

3-4 leaves of Organic Kale Blanched
4 Tablespoons Organic Hemp Powder
3 Tablespoons Organic Chia Powder
1 teaspoon Maca Powder (Fertility boosting)
1 teaspoon or less of Green Powder Stevia (depends on how sweet you prefer)
1 Banana
2 Tablespoons or more of Organic Raw Almond Butter
2 Tablespoons Organic Raw Cacao Powder (a superfood)
Organic Almond Milk (365 Brand does not contain Carrageenan)
1 teaspoon Flax Oil or 1 Tablespoon ground Flax Seeds (reduces inflammation/grind seeds in coffee grinder, fresher is best)
Add ½ -1 teaspoon Chlorella Powder (optional)

Directions:

Wash the kale and remove the leafy part, throw out the hard stem, put the leaves in the high-powered blender. If the blender is glass, add hot water to cover. If it is plastic, blanche the leaves in hot water just so they brighten in color a bit. Blend water and kale well.

Add other ingredients, except almond milk.

Add almond milk a little at a time to get desired smoothie consistency.

Add ice if needed.

*Note: Warm smoothies are good for conception. If they come out too hot, you only need to add a few ice cubes to get them a little chilled or to room temp. The idea is warm, never cold or frozen. **If you are trying for a girl**, you can omit the kale or add Goat Yogurt to the mix for variation. Substitute berries instead of banana.*

Sweet Potato Frittata
Serves 4

Ingredients:

6 large organic eggs, beaten
1 Tbs unsalted, organic butter
½ a sweet potato, small dice
½ an organic zucchini, small dice
½ cup grated Manchego Cheese
¼ tsp oregano flakes
Salt and pepper to taste

Directions:

Using a cast iron pan or medium large sauté pan, apply medium heat, and add the butter, sweet potato, and zucchini. Toss to mix in pan, and then brown well for 3 to 5 minutes. Remove from pan and set aside.

Preheat oven broiler to medium-high.

Add remaining butter to pan. On medium-low heat, add the beaten eggs to the pan. Let set for 1 to 2 minutes, then the vegetables, spices, and cheese. Let cook for another 2 to 3 minutes.

Place pan under the broiler for 2 to 3 minutes, checking every 30 seconds to avoid scorching.

Remove pan from broiler, let rest for 1 minute, slice frittata, and garnish with grated cheese and serve.

Fabulous Fertility Salad
Serves 2

Ingredients:

4 handfuls of organic mixed greens or organic baby Romaine lettuce
2 Tbs pumpkin seeds
1 tsp flax seeds
2 tsp sunflower seeds
1 organic tomato, chopped (if in season)
3 radishes, chopped (if in season)
A dash of salt

Dressing

3 Tbs organic olive oil
1 tsp apple cider vinegar
1 tsp horseradish mustard
¼ tsp oregano
¼ tsp basil

Directions:

Wash lettuce and place in large bowl. Add the seeds and tomato and radishes if in season. In a small separate bowl, mix all the ingredients for the dressing. Add the dressing to the salad and toss.

Healing Bone Broth
Serves 4

Ingredients:

2 lbs beef bones with marrow (hormone free, organic if possible)
2 stalks organic celery
3 large organic carrots
1 large organic red onion
3 cloves of garlic
2 Tbs organic apple cider vinegar

Directions:

Place all ingredients into a medium pot, cover with water and place on stove top. Turn on medium high to reach a boil. Then turn down to low heat. Allow to simmer for up to 8 hours.

Turn off heat and allow to cool on stove top for 30 minutes. Strain well, pour into glass Ball jars and refrigerate or freeze in a freezer safe container. You can drink bone broth warm or cold. You can use as a base for other soup recipes.

Gluten Free Bison Lasagna
Serves 6

Ingredients:

1 medium onion chopped
1 lb ground bison
1 jar of organic tomato puree
1 box of gluten-free lasagna noodles
4 ounces of organic goat cheese
1 cup organic spinach
2 cups Manchego cheese
1 tsp oregano

1 tsp basil
1 tsp paprika (optional)
A dash of salt

Directions:

In a cast iron pan (preferred), brown 1 chopped onion and 3 cloves of chopped garlic in butter. Remove onion and garlic, and set aside.

Brown the ground bison in butter for 3 to 5 minutes. Use high heat, and drop fist-sized pieces into pan. *Do not* over-stir. If over-stirred, the meat releases water and becomes messy and will not brown properly. Let brown, and chop up with metal spatula.

Add onion and garlic to the bison in pan, then add the tomato puree, oregano, basil, paprika (if desired) and dash of salt. Cook on medium heat for 2 to 3 minutes, then turn off. You want the sauce at medium thickness, and not watery.

Use a large, rectangular 9x11 glass baking dish or two smaller baking dishes if you want to eat one and freeze the other. Put two large spoonfuls of meat sauce in the bottom of the dish and spread to coat the surface. Add 4 tsp of water to the pan.

Add noodles in rows to cover the bottom of the pan. Top with meat sauce, but not too thickly. Add a layer of goat cheese crumbled on top of meat sauce. Add a layer of spinach. Add another layer of noodles, and press lightly down a little into the cheese.

When complete, layer the remaining meat sauce and 3 tsp of water over the top. Grate the Manchego cheese as the last layer, and cook in the oven for 30 minutes uncovered at 375 degrees.

Remove from the oven and cool 3 to 4 minutes.

Cut and serve. This dish can be reheated in oven easily.

Chicken Soup Puree
Serves 4

Ingredients:

1 ½ lbs chicken thigh meat (preferably organic, boneless, skinless)
2 cups organic chicken stock or vegetable broth
2 Tbs organic, unsalted butter
1 tsp oregano flakes
1 tsp basil flakes
3 Tbs cilantro, chopped
3 Tbs parsley, chopped
2 cloves of garlic, chopped
1 onion, medium dice
2 celery stalks, medium dice
2 cups spinach
Salt and pepper to taste
Gluten Free Crackers

Directions:

Preheat oven to 450 F. Rinse Chicken under cold water and towel dry. Place chicken thighs into a baking dish, allowing for enough room if the thighs release more liquid than expected when baked. Prepare another clean baking dish for the final dish and put to the side.

Bake chicken thighs for 18 minutes. Add 3 minutes for bone in thighs.

In a small or medium stockpot, melt the butter, and add onion, garlic, and celery. Sweat them until soft and tender for 5 to 6 minutes.

Add the stock or broth.

Remove the chicken from oven and let rest for 5 minutes. Chop chicken thighs into ¼ inch cubes and put into the stockpot.

Cook mixture on medium heat for 8 minutes. Add cilantro, parsley, basil, oregano and spinach, stirring often. Do not let boil.

Pour hot mixture into blender and run for 2 minutes. Add salt and pepper to taste. Pour into bowls and serve with gluten-free crackers.

Chicken Mexicana (Pollo Loco)
Serves 4

Ingredients:

1 ½ lbs chicken thigh meat (organic, boneless, and skinless)
2 cups organic, crushed tomatoes
2 Tbs organic, unsalted butter
2 Tbs Cholula hot sauce
1 tsp oregano flakes
1 tsp basil flakes
½ tsp chipotle powder (may omit for mild)
Salt and pepper to taste

Garnish

2 cups grated, Manchego Cheese
2 Tbs chopped Cilantro

Directions:

Preheat oven 450 F. Rinse chicken under cold water and towel dry. Place chicken thighs into a baking dish, allowing for enough room if thighs release more liquid than expected when baked. Prepare another clean baking dish for the final dish, and put to the side.

Bake chicken thighs for 18 minutes. Add 3 minutes for bone in thighs.

In a saucepan, add all other ingredients and simmer on medium heat to thicken and develop flavors. Stir often. Do not cover.

Remove chicken from oven and let rest 5 minutes. Chop chicken thighs into ¼ inch cubes and arrange in additional clean baking dish.

Cover with ¾ of the sauce (saving ¼) and grated cheese. Place under a medium to high broiler for 2 to 3 minutes.

Serve with remaining sauce. Garnish with cilantro.

Bean Enchilada
Serves 4

Ingredients:

1 can organic black beans or red kidney beans
2 Tbs organic chevre (soft goat cheese)
3 cups crushed organic tomatoes
2 Tbs unsalted, organic butter
½ tsp onion powder
1 tsp oregano flakes
1 tsp basil flakes
½ tsp chipotle powder
8 organic corn tortillas
½ cup fresh cilantro, chopped
2 cups grated Manchego Cheese
Add salt and pepper to taste

Directions:

Preheat oven 450 F. Heat beans on medium high in a sauté pan, and add butter to pan. Bring to a simmer, cook 3 to 5 minutes. Be sure to stir often to prevent scorching. Mash the beans evenly with a small whisk or large fork back, and continue to stir constantly.

Remove beans from pan and set aside in a mixing bowl. Add soft goat cheese and mix well.

In a saucepan, add tomatoes, butter, onion powder, oregano, basil, and chipotle powder. Simmer 5 to 7 minutes on medium heat. Stir often. Do not cover.

Add one third of the sauce (reserve the rest) to the beans mixture and mix well.

Soften the corn tortillas with warm water by hand. Add 3 tsp of sauce and 3 tsp water to bottom of dish. Fill with beans, roll, and arrange in a baking dish.

Cover enchiladas with the remaining sauce and grated Manchego cheese. Place in 450 F oven for 10 minutes.

Portion 2 each, garnish with chopped cilantro and serve.

Chicken Livers with Sage and Apple
Serves 4

Ingredients:

1 container Bell and Evans organic chicken livers
1 medium onion, chopped
1 pat of organic butter (for sautéing the onion)
2 organic apples, chopped
2 Tbs fresh sage

Garnish

1 apple julienne

Directions:

In a cast iron pan, brown the chopped onion in butter. Add the chicken livers after the onion has started to brown.

Let the livers begin to brown, and add the chopped apple and fresh sage. Cook until the apples are tender. The livers should cook until brown and may require chopping in pan. Do not overcook or they will become dry. Plate and garnish with julienne apple.

Curry Chicken Salad
Serves 4

Ingredients:

1 ½ lbs organic chicken thigh meat or breast (boneless and skinless)
1 organic apple (small dice)
2 stalks celery (small dice)
2 Tbs mayonnaise (safflower)
½ Tbs prepared mustard
1 tsp curry powder
½ tsp cinnamon
1 tsp honey
½ cup pistachios
Salt and pepper to taste

Directions:

Preheat oven 450 F. Rinse chicken under cold water and towel dry. Place chicken thighs into a baking dish allowing for enough room as thighs release more liquid than expected when baked. Prepare another clean baking dish for the final dish and put to the side. Bake chicken thighs for 18 minutes. Adding 3 minutes for bone in thighs. Remove chicken from oven and let rest 5 minutes. Chop chicken thighs into ¼ inch cubes and place in mixing bowl. Add to the chopped chicken, the chopped apple, celery and all remaining ingredients; be sure to mix well throughout. Portion and serve, topped with pistachios (shelled).

Sardine Pesto
Serves 2

Ingredients:

1 can of sardines (bpa free can)
3 cups fresh basil leaves
1 cup organic spinach
1 clove garlic
1 Tbs pumpkin seeds
¾ cup organic extra virgin olive oil
Salt to taste

Directions:

Place pumpkin seeds, garlic, and a pinch of salt into a mini food processor and chop well. Scrape sides. Add 1 cup basil and ¼ cup EVOO to seed/garlic blend in processor and blend through. Add 2 more cups basil and ¼ cup EVOO and blend. Add 1 cup spinach and remaining ¼ cup EVOO and blend. Taste and adjust salt as needed.

Drain sardines and place in a bowl. Add as much pesto as you like to the sardines and mix well. You can eat the sardine pesto with crackers or on gluten free toast. There will be pesto leftover to use on pasta or to use as a dip for vegetables. You can also put pesto on chicken breast or cod. It stays in the refrigerator for 2-3 days.

Black Bean Pasta with Almond Butter
Serves 4

Ingredients:

½ pound dry black bean pasta
½ cup organic red bell pepper, julienned
½ cup organic yellow bell pepper, julienned
½ cup green onion, julienned
1 cup toasted almond slices
Salt and pepper to taste

Sauce

4 Tbs organic almond butter
¼ tsp chipotle powder
1 tsp curry powder
1 tsp organic apple cider vinegar
1 tsp organic honey or agave
3 oz hot water

Directions:

Bring 8 cups salted water to boil in medium pot. Add dry pasta and cook for 6 to 7 minutes.

Drain cooked pasta, and set aside in a medium mixing bowl. Cut if necessary.

In another medium mixing bowl, add the ingredients for the sauce. Mixing with a whisk, slowly add 2 oz of hot water to the sauce, until you achieve a smooth and viscous mixture. Add remaining 1 oz of water if needed.

In a third mixing bowl, add half the sauce to half the pasta. Add half of the red and yellow julienned peppers, and half the green onion. Mix gently so as not to mash the pasta. Adjust with more sauce as needed.

It should be moist, not soupy. Serve with peppers, onion, and toasted almond slices.

Induction Eggplant Parmesan
Serves 4

Ingredients:

2 medium organic eggplants
1 red onion
2 cloves of garlic
3 Tbs olive oil
4 ounces organic crushed tomatoes
½ cup chopped fresh parsley
1 tsp oregano
1 tsp crushed red pepper
½ tsp chopped fresh / dry basil
½ tsp thyme
1 cup grated Manchego cheese
Salt and pepper to taste

Directions:

Remove most all of the dark skin from eggplant and chop the eggplant flesh in small ¼ inch squares. Place in a medium bowl and sprinkle with 2 dashes of salt, toss well.

Chop the red onion into small dice and chop the garlic. Heat a medium sauté pan to medium heat for 2 minutes, add 1 Tbs olive oil; then add the onion and garlic. Stir and sauté, allow for light browning, cooking for 4-5 minutes until tender, then remove from the pan and set aside.

Using a large sauté pan, put onto medium high heat, adding remaining olive oil to hot pan and then the eggplant. Stir well to coat eggplant with olive oil.

Let eggplant cook for 5-7 minutes, stir slightly only every 2 minutes as the eggplant browns evenly.

When desired doneness of eggplant is achieved, add the onion, garlic, tomatoes and all remaining spices and herbs to the eggplant in a large rectangular dish. Sprinkle with Manchego cheese, add salt and pepper to taste and place in heated oven at 375 for 5-10 minutes until cheese melts. Serve warm.

Roasted Onions and Garlic
Serves 4

Ingredients:

2 medium red onions
2 heads of garlic
2 Tbs avocado oil
Salt to taste

Directions:

Preheat oven to 375 F. In a medium baking dish, add the oil and coat the bottom of the dish well. Cut the onion and garlic in half, cross ways (top/bottom) and place each half face side down into the baking dish.

Bake for 25 minutes. Remove from oven, salt and let cool enough to eat. Sometimes the onion may need longer, if so remove roasted garlic and add 5 minutes to the onion until desired doneness. Serve with any dish ½ onion person and ½ head of garlic person. More or less if desired.

Foods to Avoid

Breakfast bars (high in sugar and carbs)
Boxed or frozen meals (high sodium and too many preservatives)
Chips or snacks with no nutritional value
Lunch meat and deli meat (high in nitrates)
Fish high in mercury
Dairy with rGBH hormones and GMOs
Hormone-laden meats and chicken
Soy and soy products, soy oil
Canola oil
Sugar
Sushi
Margarine and fake butter spreads
Trans fats
Hydrogenated fats
Foods with food coloring
Artificial sweeteners
Sugar, which includes cakes, baked items, candy, donuts, etc.
Caffeine (coffee and some teas)
Processed foods
Fast foods
Fried Foods
Canned foods (with the exception BPA-free canned beans)
Microwave popcorn (perfluorooctanoic acid exposure in bag lining)
Soda
Sports Drinks (contains sugar and chemicals)
Alcohol
Erythritol (ingredient in some sugar free sports drinks)
Carrageenan(ingredient in alternative milks and other proucts)
Too many cold or raw foods
Gluten
Gluten free products which are not Non-GMO(just because it is gluten
free does not mean it is GMO free)

REFERENCES

Adams, Stephen. "Forget BMI, Just measure your waist and height' say Scientists," May 12, 2012, Telegraph.co.uk, © 2014 Telegraph Media Group Limited.

Anderson, Virginia. "Case Study: Infertility and Reiki Healing," PositiveHealth.com, originally listed in Fertility, originally published in issue 171 - June 2010, © 2011 Compass Internet Ltd.

Barton, Dalene. "Defective MTHFR Gene Linked to Fertility and Pregnancy Struggles," ©2007-2014 The Natural Fertility Company.

Betts, Debra. "Natural Pain Relief Techniques for Childbirth Using Acupressure, Promoting A Natural Labour and Partner Involvement," © 2003 Debra Betts.

Blossom Orange. "Pineapple and IVF Success- It's all about Embryo Implantation," BlossomClinic.net, © 2013 Blossom Orange.

Campbell, Leah. "Using Bromelain to Encourage Implantation – One Pineapple Slice at a Time," Natural-fertility-info.com, ©2007-2014 The Natural Fertility Company.

Connett, Michael. "Fluoride's Effect On Fetal Brain," August 2012, Fluoridealert.org, ©2012 Fluoride Action Network.

Cunha, John P. "Mercury Poisoning Facts," April 2014, Medicinenet. com, © 1996-2014 MedicineNet, Inc.

Davis, Jeanie Lerche. Reviewed by; Dr. Charlotte E. Grayson Mathis, Pool Water Risky During Pregnancy,", WebMD.com Health News, ©2005-2014 WebMD, LLC.

Doheny, Kathleen, Editor: Dr. Louise Chang. "Deciding Baby's Sex, Can Diet, Timing, and Changing Body Chemistry Really Determine the Sex of Your Baby," WebMD.com, © 2005-2014 WebMD, LLC.

Dr. Dittmann. "Fluoride Linked to Infertility, Birth Defects and Low IQ," Sept. 3, 2012, NaturalHealth365.com, © 2014 Natural Health 365.

Dr. Rubin Naiman PhD, IIN Conference, Lecture, May 17 2014, NYC New York.

Faith, Norah. "Diet to Conceive a Boy," EHow.com, © 1999-2014 Demand Media, Inc.

Fleming, Dawn. "Reiki and Fertility: Getting the Body in Balance to Increase Fertility and Pregnancy Odds," October 23, 2013, NaturalNews.com, © 2014 Natural News Network.

Greenberg, Dr. James A and Stacey J Bell. "Multivitamin Supplementation During Pregnancy: Emphasis on Folic Acid and l-Methylfolate," © 2011 MedReviews®, LLC.

Greger, Dr. Michael. "Foods With Natural Melatonin," April 3, 2014, Nutritionfacts.org, © 2014 NutritionFacts.org.

Haiken, Melanie. "5 Surprising Foods That Help You Sleep," June 30, 2012, © 2014 Forbes.com, Inc.

Herrington, Diana. "15 Amazing Benefits of Ghee," Apr 143, 2014, Care2.com, © 2014.

John, Esther M., David A. Savitz and Carl M. Shy. "Spontaneous Abortions among Cosmetologists," © 2014 International Society for Environmental Epidemiology, Lippincott Williams & Wilkins.

Kain, Erica. "Trying to Get Pregnant? 10 Proven Sperm Killers," Health.com, © 2014 Health Media Ventures, Inc.

Kent, Linda Tarr. "Tyrosine & Sleep," Aug 16, 2013, Livestrong.com, © 2014 Demand Media, Inc.

Lee, Mi Kyeong, and Soon Bok Chang, and Duck-Hee Kang. "Effects of SP6 Acupressure on Labor Pain and Length of Delivery Time in Women During Labor," March 9, 2005, The Journal of Alternative and Complementary Medicine. December 2004, 10(6): 959-965.

Lepisto, Christine."10 Beauty Products You Must Ditch During Pregnancy," March 18, 2010, Treehugger.com, © 2014 MNN Holding Company, LLC

McDermott, Nick. "Mothers Who Swim During Pregnancy," Sept. 1, 2013, Dailymail.uk.co, © **2013.**

McNally, Shelagh. "Is your House Toxic? 6 Household Cleaning Chemicals You Should Avoid," Greenlivingonline.com, © 2014 Green Living Enterprises Inc.

Minahan, Monique. "Maya Massage: A Healing Practice Every Woman Should Know," Jan 14, 2013, Huffingtonpost.com, ©2014 TheHuffingtonPost.com, Inc.

Noorlander, AM, and JPM Geraedts, JBM Melissen "Female Gender Pre-Selection by Maternal Diet in Combination with Timing of Sexual Intercourse – a Prospective Study," August 2010, RBMonline.com, © 2010 Reproductive Healthcare Ltd., Published by Elsevier Ltd.

Oz, Daphne. "Arvigo Maya Fertility Massage: More Than a Belly Rub," March 17, 2010, Oprah.com, © 2014 HARPO PRODUCTIONS, INC.

Patel, Arti. "Best Foods For Iron: 20 Foods Packed With Iron," Nov 15 2012, TheHuffingtonPost.Ca, ©2014 TheHuffingtonPost.com, Inc.

Renter, Elizabeth. "8 Foods to Naturally Increase Melatonin for Better Sleep," Aug. 20, 2013, © 2014 Conscious Life News.

Rex. "Diabetes and Young Living Essential Oil Products," September 17, 2012, TheOcoteaNewsletter.com, © 2011 The Ocotea Newsletter, LLC.

Riley, Ellen Ruoff and Stuart Robbins. Medical Editor: Dr. George Krucik, "The Best Air-Purifying Plants," February 27, 2013, Healthline. com, © 2005 - 2014 Healthline Networks, Inc.

Rodriguez, Dr. Hethir. "How to Increase Your Egg Health in 90 Days, "Natural-Fertility-Info.com, ©2007-2014 The Natural Fertility Company.

Rufus, Anneli. "Can Food Make You Infertile? Foods to Eat and Avoid," TheDailyBeast.com, © 2014 The Daily Beast Company LLC.

Rush, Colleen. "8 Beauty No-Nos When You're Preg-O, Which ingredients you should cut out of your regimen," TotalBeauty.com, ©2007 - 2014 Total Beauty Media, Inc.

Sandbeck, Ellen. *Organic Housekeeping.* ©2006 Simon and Schuster.

St-Onge, Elina. "You Have The Right To Know: 17 Chemicals To Avoid In Cosmetic And Personal Care Products," April 10, 2012, © 2014 Collective-Evolution.com.

Stöppler, Melissa Conrad. Medical Editor: Dr. William C. Shiel Jr., "Polycystic Ovarian Syndrome (PCOS, POS, POD, Stein-Leventhal

Syndrome)," article, page 5, Medicinenet.com, ©1996-2014 MedicineNet, Inc.

Todd, Dr. Nivin. "Can Labor Be Induced Naturally?" May 25, 2014, WebMD.com, © 2014 WebMD, LLC.

Wang, Peggy. "10 Common Beauty Products You Shouldn't Be Putting On Your Skin," Sept. 19, 2013, BuzzFeed.com, © 2014 BuzzFeed, Inc.

Weber, Kathryn. "Feng Shui Fertility — Six Ways to Create More Baby Chi," May 15, 2013, RedLotusLetter.com, © 2014 Kathryn Weber.

Weber, Kathryn. "Feng Shui for Fertility," ConceiveOnline.com, © 1997-2014 BabyCenter, LLC.

Wright, Hillary. "The PCOS Diet Plan- A Natural Approach to Health for Women with Polycystic Ovary Syndrome," © 2012-2013 Pcosdietsupport.com.

Acupuncture.com/education/points/gallbladder/gb21.htm

AnnBoroch.com

"Arvigo Maya Fertility Massage; A Fertility-Enhancing Massage, with No Chocolate or Champagne," Feb. 11, 2010, Well+Good.com, © 2014 Well+Good LLC.

Arvigotherapy.com

"The Benefits of Reiki While Pregnant," May 30, 2013, Mumazine Mums, Mumazine.com, ©2014 Mumazine.

Blogtalkradio.com/haveababy/2013/05/08/have-a-baby-radio

"Celiac Disease Gluten Sensitivity and Your Fertility," article, TheAFA. org, ©2014 The American Fertility Association.

Celiacdiseasecenter.columbia.edu, © 2014 Celiac Disease Center at Columbia University.

"Conception and Fertility-The Male Reproductive Cycle," defined, PAMF.org, © 2014 Palo Alto Medical Foundation.

"Diet Tips- PCOS and Gluten," article, PCOSDietSupport.com, © 2012-2013 www.pcosdietsupport.com.

"Does Eating Pineapple Help Implantation? Fertility Wonder Foods, Separating Myth from Fact," FertilityAfter40.com, © 2013.

Drjennifermercier.com

DrNaiman.com, © 2014 Dr. Rubin Naiman.

"Endometriosis- Basic Symptoms," defined, Mayoclinic.org, © 1998-2014 Mayo Foundation for Medical Education and Research.

"Endometriosis," defined, Medicinenet.com, ©1996-2014 MedicineNet, Inc.

"Endometriosis," defined, Drweil.com, © 2014 Weil Lifestyle, LLC.

"Exposure to Chlorine In Pregnancy," UK Teratology Information Service, UKTIS.org, © 2012 UKTIS.

"Facts About Chlorine," The Center for Disease Control and Prevention, © 2013 BT.CDC.Gov.

Fertilitychicago.org

"Frequently Asked Questions," The Bradley Method, Bradleybirth.com, © 2014 AAHCC.

"Health Topics- Endometriosis," article, PCRM.org, © 2014 The Physicians Committee.

"The Health Effects of Wood Smoke," Environment and Human Health, Inc., EHHI.org, © EHHI.

"Hidden Dangers of Pregnancy Fitness and Swimming," DivineCaroline. com, © 2013 Divine Caroline.

Holisticdental.org

©2014 TheHuffingtonPost.com, Inc.

"HypnoBirthing- The Mongan Method," Hypnobirthing.com, © 2000 - 2012 HypnoBirthing Institute.

"Increase Milk Supply with Lactogenic Foods, Foods that Increase Milk Supply," © 2014 breastfeeding-problems.com.

"Increasing Iron in Your Diet During Pregnancy," Clevelandclinic.org, © 1995-2014 Cleveland Clinic.

"Natural Ways to Induce Labor," WhattoExpect.com, © 2013 What to Expect, LLC.

"Pituitary," defined, UCLA.edu, © 2006 The Regents of the University of California.

"Pregnancy Tumor," defined, SimplestepsDental.com, © 2002-2014 Aetna, Inc.

"Pregnancy Wellness- Mercury Levels in Fish," article, AmericanPregnancy.org, © 2014 American Pregnancy Association.

"Safe Skin Care During Pregnancy," article, Babycenter.ca, © 1997-2014 BabyCenter LLC.

"Stress and Infertility, Doctors offer insights on how daily stress can disrupt fertility -- and how relaxation can help," WedMD.com, ©2005-2014 WebMD, LLC.

©2014 www.toxichotseatmovie.com

"What Is A Doula?" DONA.org, © 2013 DONA International.

"What's New and Beneficial About Quinoa," WHFoods.com, © 2001-2014 The George Mateljan Foundation.

"Why Consider Delayed Cord Clamping?" Oct. 11, 2012, Science ofMom.com, © 2013 Science of Mom.

"Worst Cleaners: EWG's List Of Most Harmful Cleaning Products For Your Home," Sept. 10, 2012

Permission for use of personal quote: Catalina Rivera Permission for use of Author Photo: Bradford Rogne

NOTES

[1] http://www.scientificamerican.com/article/chemicals-umbilical-cord-blood

[2] http://www.telegraph.co.uk/health/healthnews/9260091/Forget-BMI-just-measure-your-waist-and-height-say-scientists.html

[3] http://time.com/14407/the-hidden-dangers-of-skinny-fat/

[4] http://www.everydayhealth.com/gestational-diabetes/oral-medications-for-gestational-diabetes.aspx

[5] http://www.celiaccentral.org/newlydiagnosed/Related-Conditions/Infertility/41/

[6] http://natural-fertility-info.com/preventing-miscarriage

[7] http://www.westonaprice.org/health-topics/diet-for-pregnant-and-nursing-mothers/

[8] http://en.wikipedia.org/wiki/Bottom_feeder carp, and sturgeon

[9] http://www.stopthethyroidmadness.com/mthfr/

[10] http://www.ncbi.nlm.nih.gov/pmc/articles/PMC3250974/

[11] http://www.doctoroz.com/videos/does-vitamin-d-prevent-fibroids

[12] http://www.medpagetoday.com/OBGYN/Pregnancy/38113

[13] http://www.webmd.com/food-recipes/news/20130129/brominated-vegetable-oil-qa; http://en.wikipedia.org/wiki/Brominated_vegetable_oil

[14] http://www.thenibble.com/reviews/nutri/matter/organic-coffee3.asp

[15] http://toxnet.nlm.nih.gov/cpdb/pdfs/handbook.pesticide.toxicology.pdf

[16] http://www.cdc.gov/features/dssleep/; http://guardianlv.com/2014/02/sleep-disorders-top-4-that-make-70-million-suffer/

[17] http://www.forbes.com/sites/melaniehaiken/2012/06/30/5-surprising-foods-that-help-you-sleep/

[18] http://www.collective-evolution.com/2012/04/10/you-have-the-right-to-know-17-chemicals-to-avoid-in-cosmetic-and-personal-care-products/

[19] http://safecosmetics.org/section.php?id=75

[20] http://www.collective-evolution.com/2012/04/10/you-have-the-right-to-know-17-chemicals-to-avoid-in-cosmetic-and-personal-care-products/

[21] http://www.collective-evolution.com/2013/09/14/attention-deodorant-users-new-studies-link-aluminum-to-breast-cancer/

22   http://www.epa.gov/dfe/pubs/garment/ctsa/factsheet/ctsafaq.htm#1

23   http://www.cancer.org/cancer/cancercauses/othercarcinogens/
generalinformationaboutcarcinogens/known-and-probable-human-carcinogens

24   www.toxichotseatmovie.com

25   http://www.blossomclinic.net/2013/05/30/pineapple-and-embryo-
implantation-ivf-success/

26   http://nutgourmet.wordpress.com/2010/04/30/brazil-nuts-the-dr-jekyll-
and-mr-hyde-of-the-nut-world/;

27   http://diaryofayummymummyinwaiting.co.uk/old-wives-tales/

28   http://www.babyzone.com/getting-pregnant/how-to-get-pregnant/
foods-to-boost-fertility_88525#gallery/brazil-nuts
http://www.webmd.com/baby/news/20080423/
ominous-rise-in-prepregnancy-diabetes

29   http://www.huffingtonpost.com/intent/maya-massage_b_2388751.html

30   http://www.huffingtonpost.com/intent/maya-massage_b_2388751.html

31   http://wellandgood.com/2010/02/11/a-fertility-enhancing-massage-with-no-
chocolate-or-champagne/

32   http://www.webmd.com/baby/inducing-labor-naturally-can-it-be-done

33   http://www.positivehealth.com/article/fertility/case-study-
infertility-and-reiki-healing

34   http://www.naturalnews.com/042614_Reiki_fertility_energy_therapy.
html#ixzz38g2UxBTO

35   http://www.mumazine.com/article/2013/05/30/benefits-reiki-while-pregnant

36   http://www.mayoclinic.org/healthy-living/pregnancy-week-by-week/in-depth/
prenatal-yoga/art-20047193

37   http://www.bradleybirth.com/faqs.aspx

38   http://www.hypnobirthing.com/

39   http://www.dona.org/mothers/

40   http://www.medicalnewstoday.com/articles/263181.php

41   http://scienceofmom.com/2012/10/11/why-consider-delayed-cord-clamping/

42   Aromatherapy: Essential Oils in Practice, Jane Buckle PHD, RN

43   http://www.sciencedirect.com/science/book/9780443072369

44   http://www.med-health.net/Cinnamon-Powder.html

45   http://en.wikipedia.org/wiki/Freedom_%28philosophy%29

46   http://en.wikipedia.org/wiki/Morality
http://en.wikipedia.org/wiki/Waldorf_education

47   http://www.medicaldaily.com/microwaves-are-bad-you-5-reasons-why-
microwave-oven-cooking-harming-your-health-250145; http://articles.mercola.
com/sites/articles/archive/2010/05/18/microwave-hazards.aspx

HOSPITAL BIRTH GO BAG CHECKLIST!
FOR MOM

Nursing tops, tanks or bras (cotton, natural fiber, comfortable style and long sleeve if you get cold) (3, or more if scheduled C- section which will mean more days in hospital)

Black or dark cotton leggings or loose maternity pants that are comfortable to sleep in (3)

Boy shorts or comfy panties in black or dark color...won't stain

Socks for cold feet (3)

Slippers you don't mind throwing out or can wash(dirty hospital floors)

Robe

Outfit to leave the hospital or take a picture in

Mug for tea and Traditional Medicinal Mother's milk tea.(hospital may have Styrofoam or plastic)

Glass bowl, spoon and gluten free instant oatmeal(you will become more hungry as you nurse...ravenous in my case, also oatmeal promotes breastmilk production

Ipod with hypnobirthing affirmations, comforting music for you and baby to bond, I preferred Eckhar Tolle's "Music to Quiet the Mind" for all my births and baby bonding time

Essential Oils and diffuser to set the mood and calm

Birthing ball if needed

Coconut water, nuts, applesauce, or whatever snacks you prefer…maybe a friend can bring you organic meals! Use caution when eating at first..some foods can irritate baby and are common allergens when breastfeeding.

Cosmetics, shampoo/conditioner, soap, toothpaste, toothbrush, comb/hairbrush, moisturizer, Earth mama angel baby nipple cream, coconut oil

Medications or vitamins you take(hospital vitamins are not organic)

Organic chlorine free maternity pads or heavy flow pads

Reusable nursing pads which are organic or Bamboobies

Camera, phone, phone charger, camera charger

Your own pillow and pillowcase. If you are extremely sensitive…bring your own sheets.

Nursing pillow which is of safe materials/organic cover

FOR BABY

3 blankets to swaddle the baby that are ORGANIC(We used the hospital blankets at first, baby had a rash, I pulled my blankets out of the suitcase and rash went away! Hospital linens are cleaned with harsh detergents.)

3 Organic tops that are easy to open with snaps in the front…not ones you have to pull over the head and snap like a onesie. (Baby will have a clamp on umbilical cord, you will be checking diapers and need easy access.)

3 Organic Pants without feet(Baby will have a moniter for protection and it may not fit if there are feet in the pants.

3 pair of organic socks(they will most likely fall off and baby will be swaddled to keep feet warm anyway, but just in case)

3 pair of organic mittens if the tops do not have the built in covers for the hands

3 organic hats to keep the baby's head warm

Honest Newborn Diapers and Honest Wipes or size 1 if you know the baby will be larger

Earth Mama Angel Baby Unscented Shampoo/Body wash for baby's first bath in the hospital (don't use the hospital soap!!!toxic!!)

Honest Diaper Cream just in case..I just put breastmilk on rashes or irritations in the first weeks or coconut oil.

Going home outfit in Organic cotton preferred!

Carseat in safe fabric without flame retardants

For Husband or Partner

3 boxers, 3 tshirts, 3 pants, 3 pairs of socks, slippers that can be tossed or washed

3 pair of sleeping pants(nurse will be in and out of room all night to check on you and the baby…no sleeping in the buff)

One going home outfit or outfit for pictures

Favorite snacks

Toiletries, razer, shave cream, toothbrush, toothpaste, comb/brush

RESOURCES

Celiac Disease-www.celiaccentral.org

Campaign for Safe Cosmetics-www.safecosmetics.org

Doula Association-www.dona.org

Dr. Mercola-www.mercola.com-natural health

Environmental Working Group-www.ewg.org-lists and researches safe products/foods

Green Pasture-www.greenpasture.org-fish oil and related products

Holistic Dental Association-www.holisticdental.org

Ina May Gaskin Midwife-www.inamaygaskin.com

La Leche League-www.llli.org-breastfeeding support

Mercier Therapy-www.merciertherapy.com-to support conception with massage

Mongon Hypnobirthing-www.hypnobirthing.com

Gene mutation MTHFR-www.mthfr.net

Multiple Sclerosis- www.annboroch.com

Mountain Rose Herbs-www.mountainroseherbs.com

Non-GMO Foods-www.nongmoproject.com

www.nuts.com

Shaklee-www.shaklee.com-cleaning products

Young Living- wendieaston.marketingscents.com-essential oils

Weston A. Price-www.westonaprice.org

Waldorf-www.whywaldorfworks.com

RECOMMENDED READING

Boroch, Ann, CNC *The Candida Cure, Yeast, Fungus & Your Health*, Los Angeles: Quintessential Healing Publishing, 2009

Dancy, Rahima Baldwin, *You Are Your Child's First Teacher*, Berkeley: Ten Speed Press, 1989

Green, Peter H.R., MD, *Celiac Disease: A Hidden Epidemic*, William Morrow, 2010

Hyman, Dr. Mark, *The Blood Sugar Solution*, New York: Little Brown and Company, 2014

Miller, Lorraine, *From Gratitude to Bliss*, Balboa Press, *2014*

Payne, Kim John, *Simplicity Parenting: Using the Extraordinary Power of Less to Raise Calmer, Happier, and More Secure Kids*, New York: Ballantine Books, 2009

Sears, William, MD and Martha Sears, RN, *The Baby Sleep Book: The Complete Guide to a Good Night's Rest for the Whole Family*, New York: Little Brown and Company, 2005

Sears, William, MD and Martha Sears, RN, *The Attachment Parenting Book: A Common Sense Guide to Understanding and Nurturing Your Baby*, Little Brown and Company 2001

DOCUMENTARIES ON HEALTH

The Business of Being Born (2008)

Bought (2015)

Doctored (2012)

Genetic Roulette: The Gamble of Our Lives (2012)

The Greater Good (2011)

The Human Experiment (2013)

Hungry for Change(2013)

Toxic Hot Seat (2013)

Unacceptable Levels (2012)

The War on Wheat (2015)

INDEX

ABOUT THE AUTHOR

As a Certified Holistic Health Coach, lecturer, author, and HypnoBirthing practitioner, Wendie Aston teaches others an organic way of life. Her long time passion for eating organic and living eco-friendly lead her on this journey. She has been researching various ways of making non-toxic choices for her home and lifestyle for over a decade. Green on the Scene, her blog, has been educating people on all things GREEN since 2010. She is available for speaking engagements, workshops and private coaching. She is also a Young Living Independent Distributor teaching people about the uses of essential oils. She currently lives on Long Island, NY with her husband and 3 children.

www.greenonthescene.blogspot.com
Green on the Scene on Facebook
Young Living Distributor #1669862
www.wendieaston.marketingscents.com/go/ms-oils